Issues in Flap Surgery

http://dx.doi.org/10.5772/66023

Edited by Sherif Amr

Contributors

Merdan Serin, Ashraf Khater, Adel Fathi, Hosam Ghazy, Goktekin Tenekeci, Masaki Fujioka, Wenceslao M Calonge, Gianluca Sapino, Yueh-Bih Tang, Jingzhi Yang, Juliane C. Finke, Marius Bredell, Michael O. Glocker, Uwe Von Fritschen, Francisco Martinez Martinez, Maria Llanos Guerrero Navarro, Juan García Navarro, Alberto Gimenez Ros, Alba Izquierdo Robledano

First published in London, United Kingdom, 2018 by IntechOpen

IntechOpen is the global imprint of INTECHOPEN LIMITED, registered in England and Wales, registration number: 11086078, The Shard, 25th floor, 32 London Bridge Street

London, SE19SG – United Kingdom

Printed in Croatia

British Library Cataloguing-in-Publication Data

A catalogue record for this book is available from the British Library

Additional hard copies can be obtained from orders@intechopen.com

Issues in Flap Surgery, Edited by Sherif Amr

p. cm.

Print ISBN 978-1-78923-012-3

Online ISBN 978-1-78923-013-0

For EU product safety concerns:
IN TECH d.o.o., Prolaz Marije Krucifikse Kozulić 3, 51000 Rijeka, Croatia,
info@intechopen.com or visit our website at intechopen.com.

Meet the editor

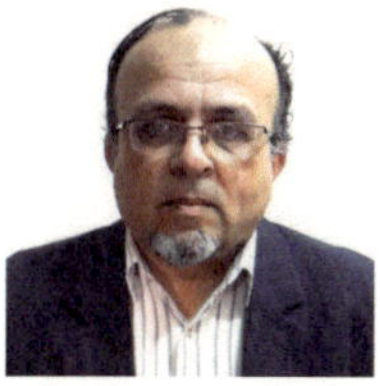

Sherif Amr is currently a professor of Orthopedics and Traumatology at the Faculty of Medicine, Cairo University. He is an orthopedic surgeon, a hand surgeon, a microsurgeon, a peripheral nerve surgeon, and a brachial plexus surgeon. He was born on March 31, 1961. He received his MBBCh degree from the Cairo University in 1985, MSc degree in 1989, and MD (PhD) degree in 1996. He further graduated from the Faculty of Law, Cairo University, with a bachelor's degree in Law in 2000. He worked as an intern at the Faculty of Medicine, Cairo University, 1986; an orthopedic resident at the Department of Orthopedics, Cairo University, 1978–1990; an assistant lecturer at the Department of Orthopedics, Cairo University, 1990–1996; a lecturer at the same department, 1996–2001; and an assistant professor, 2001–2006, before being appointed as a full professor in 2006. Additionally, he worked as a visiting resident at the Department of Plastic Surgery Medical School Hannover (MHH), Germany, and a research worker at the Department of Engineering Biomechanics, Technical University Hamburg/Harburg, 1997. He was the director of the animal research facility at the Faculty of Medicine, Cairo University from 2007 to 2011. His main research interests are microsurgery, hand surgery, surgery of peripheral nerves, brachial plexus surgery, neuroscience, and experimental orthopedic biomechanics.

Contents

Preface

The development of flap surgery parallels the increasing complexity of soft-tissue defects needing reconstruction. Random and pedicled flaps as well as free muscle and fasciocutaneous flaps have helped to reconstruct single soft-tissue defects. The multiplicity of defects needing reconstruction and donor-site morbidity in addition to tailored reconstruction have called for a revision of flap concepts in favor of perforator flaps. Unfortunately, we are faced with increasingly complex reconstructive issues. New reconstructive techniques, such as the Ilizarov method, have made orthopedic reconstruction after high energy and complex trauma possible. Revision surgeries after tumor resection and plastic surgery have brought about soft-tissue defects associated with extensive fibrosis and necrosis. As a result, previously non-salvageable limbs have been salvaged. The reconstructive surgeons are faced with the following situations: multiple soft-tissue defects, extensive fibrosis, possibility of major vessel loss, and possibility of damage of several perforators. In this book, we address some of these problems. In the basic science section, Dr. Glocker Michael demonstrates how plasma cytokine and growth factor profiling during free flap transplantation may aid in minimizing ischemia reperfusion injury during free flap planning. Dr. Serin Merdan provides many versatile experimental rat flap models. The principles and techniques of perforator flaps are revised by Dr. Tenekeci Goktekin. Dr. Fujioka Masaki contributes two important articles on the applications of perforator flaps: the application of free flow-through anterolateral thigh flap for reconstruction of soft-tissue defects requiring vascularization and emergent or early flap resurfacing for bone-exposing wounds of Gustilo-Anderson IIIB and C fractures. Special situations need a special consideration. Prof. Tang Yueh-Bih illustrates his experience in reconstructing bone and soft-tissue defects for mandibular implant failure. Dr. Martinez Martinez Francisco provides a valuable review on hand flaps. Dr. Khater Ashraf demonstrates his experience using omental flaps in breast reconstruction. Hypospadias surgery has always been a challenge because of difficult flap planning and subsequent necrosis and fibrosis. Dr. Calonge Wenceslao contributes an article on overview of hypospadias surgery.

Sherif Amr
Cairo University, Egypt

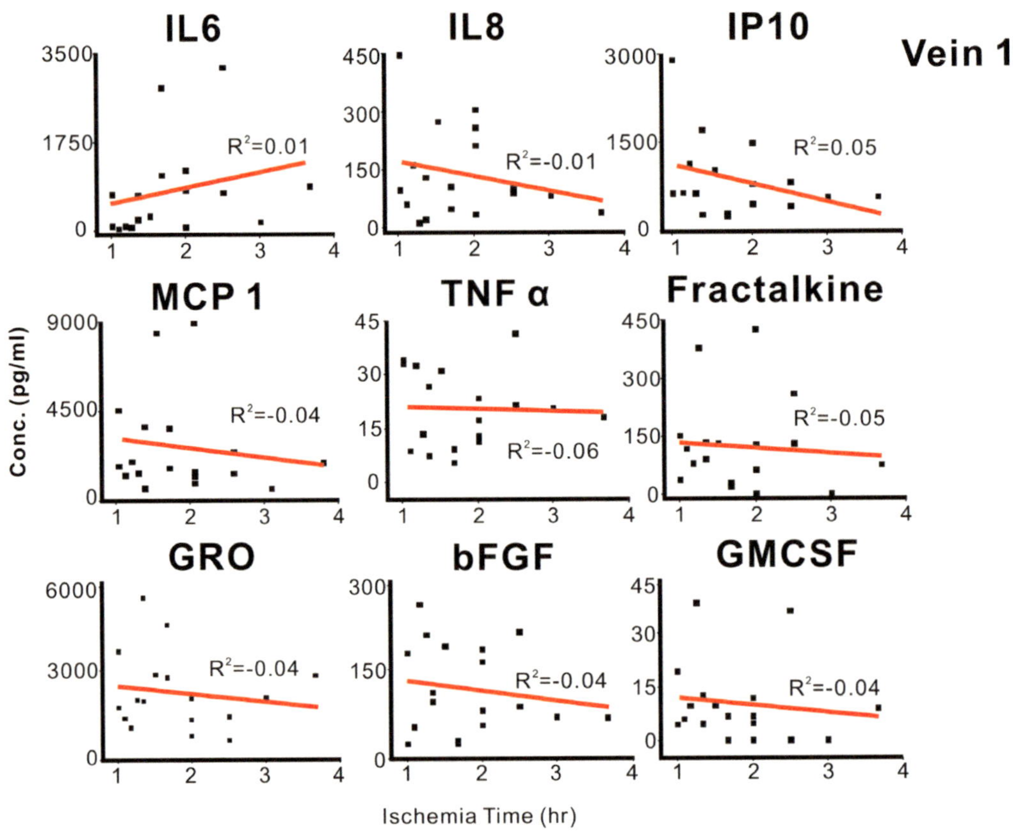

Figure 1. Linear regression plots for group I proteins between ischemia time and protein concentrations of all patients' Vein 1 samples. Trend lines are shown. R^2 values are given.

GMCSF, TNFα, Fractalkine, bFGF, and IL8 were found in low concentrations (below 500 pg/mL; colored black in **Figure 3**), whereas IP10 was found with intermediate concentration (500 pg/mL < protein concentration < 1000 pg/mL; colored dark grey) in all three sampling time points (artery, Vein 1, and Vein 2). MCP1 and GRO were present in highest concentrations (above 1000 pg/mL; colored bright grey) in most samples of all three sampling time points. Interestingly, IL6 was found to change in concentration from low in artery to intermediate in both, Vein 1 and Vein 2 samples, and prompted to analyze protein concentration differences between sampling time points.

2.3. Analysis of individual protein concentration dynamics

To investigate expression differences between the sampling time points for each patient, ratios between the respective protein concentrations were calculated. Quotient I (artery/artery), quotient II (Vein 1/artery), and quotient III (Vein 2/artery) showed individual values for all three time points in a normalized fashion. Combining these quotients, values with straight lines visualized "up" and "down" and/or "no" changes, respectively. From all investigated protein concentrations, a "dynamic" expression was observed for IL6 and IL8 in individual patients.

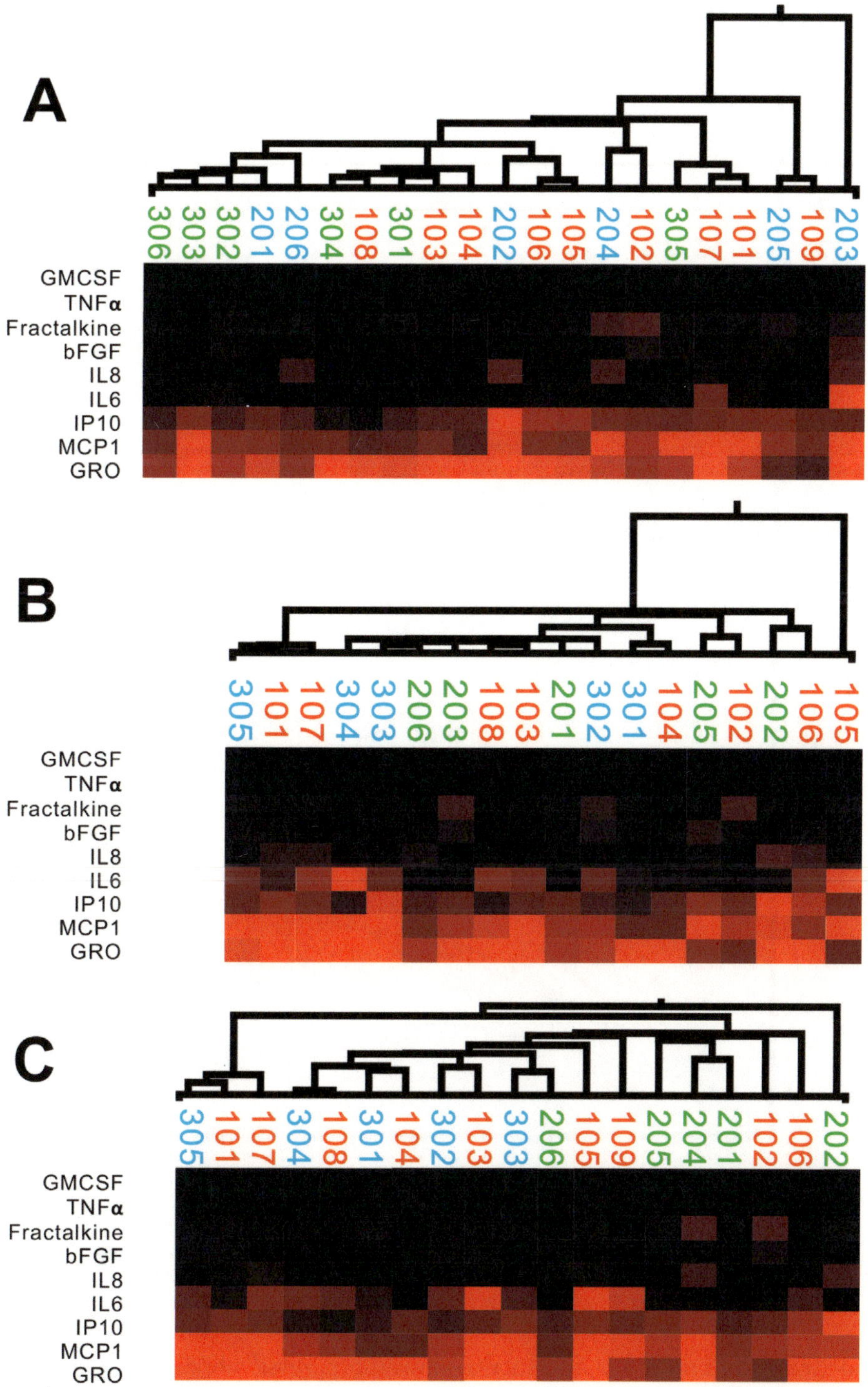

Figure 2. Hierarchical clustering analysis of protein concentrations from artery (A), Vein 1 (B), and Vein 2 (C) plasma samples of flap transplant patients. Proteins are indicated on the left. Patient IDs (**Table 1**) are given between the dendrogram and the heat map illustration. Grey scales indicate protein concentration: black—low, dark grey—medium, bright grey—high.

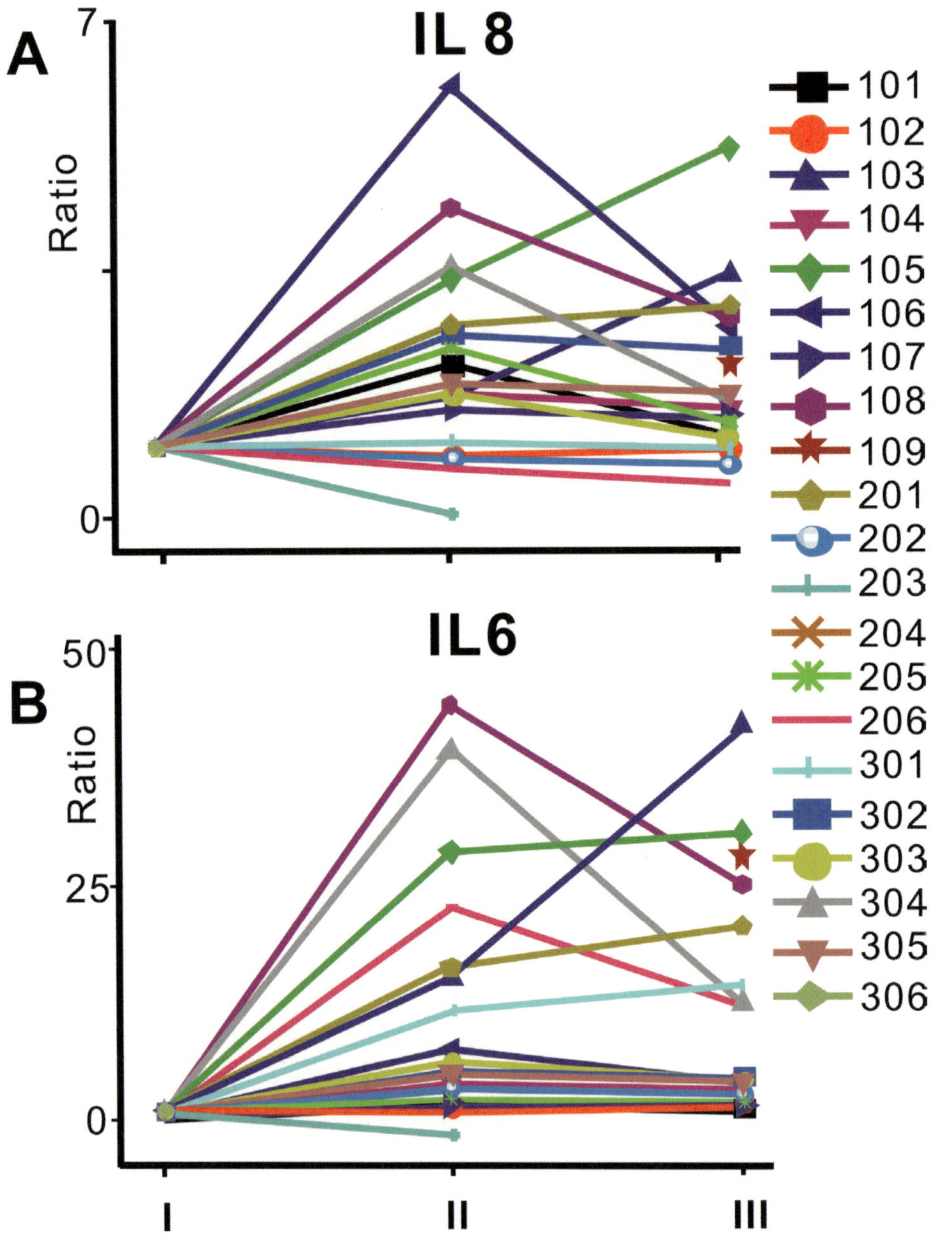

Figure 3. Line graphs of concentration ratios from 21 patients (58 plasma samples) for IL8 (A) and IL6 (B). Individual ratios were calculated from protein concentrations: I: artery/artery, II: Vein 1/artery, and III: Vein 2/artery. Patient IDs (**Table 1**) and respective symbols are shown at the right.

Nearly all line graphs for IL8 in all patients showed progression lines that were quite similar to each other (**Figure 3A**). The dominant protein concentration change profile of IL8 followed a rapid "up-down" trend. A few patients in the IL8 group (104, 107, 201, 302, and 305) represented a "slow dynamic," i.e., an "up-no" trend. Interestingly, line graphs for IL6 of most

http://dx.doi.org/10.5772/intechopen.70054

patients followed a related progression (**Figure 3B**) as well. The dominant protein profile for IL6 followed an "up-no" trend. Noteworthy, with a few patients (104, 106, 108, 206, and 304) from the IL6 group, a "fast dynamics" of protein concentration changes ("up-down" trend) was observed.

2.4. Subgroup analysis of different free flap tissue groups

Subgroup analysis of protein profiles with respect to different transplant types was performed to check whether the trend of the general protein concentration profiles of either IL6 or IL8 was found consistently in the clinical subgroups. In each of the three transplant groups (**Figure 4**), the "up-no" trend of IL6 was dominant (10 cases), followed by the "up-down" trend (5 cases).

Notably, the PPS data in the osteo-cutaneous group showed very large differences of IL6 concentrations between the pre-ischemia time point (artery) and the second post-ischemia time point (Vein 2) in patients 103, 105, and 109 ("up-no" trend). In patient 103, the difference was 2398.4 pg/mL; in patient 105, it was 3320.68 pg/mL; and in patient 109, 1549.19 pg/mL. These three patients experienced the longest ischemia times during operation (**Table 1**). Patient 109 developed a venous thrombosis after venous anastomosis, so a revision of the anastomosis with thrombectomy and an interposition of a vein graft became necessary.

Of note, in the skin flap group, the pre-ischemia value (artery) of IL6 was higher in patients with clinical conspicuities compared to the other patients. In patient 305, the pre-ischemia IL6 concentration was 144.98 pg/mL, and in patient 302, it was 147.34 pg/mL. In the other patients of this group, the pre-ischemia IL6 concentrations were much lower and the mean was 52.15 pg/mL. Patient 305 developed an intraoperative thrombosis of the artery after venous anastomosis. In patient 302, ischemia time was the longest in the whole group with 150 min.

In case of IL8, the "up-down" trend was dominant (five cases) in both, the osteo-cutaneous group (**Figure 5A**) and the cutaneous group (**Figure 5C**), followed by the "up-no" trend (four cases). Only the muscle group seemed to behave different (**Figure 5B**). Here, no dominant trend could be defined, but "up-down" cases were present.

Again, when looking at the PPS data also in the muscle group, the two patients (patients 202 and 203) with clinical conspicuities were standing out by looking at the concentrations of IL6 and additionally of IL8. In these patients, the pre-ischemia values (artery) of both, IL6 and IL8, were significantly higher than those of the other patients. The IL6 concentration of patient 202 was 30.47 pg/mL and that of patient 203 was 7064.18 pg/mL. Although both values were very different, they were much higher than the mean concentration of the other patients which was 12.81 pg/mL. Similarly, the IL8 concentration of patient 202 was 530.33 pg/mL and that of patient 203 was 477.09 pg/mL. These concentrations were again much higher than the mean (202.16 pg/mL) of all other patients in this group. Patient 202 suffered from partial flap necrosis, whereas patient 203 developed an intraoperative venous thrombosis after venous anastomosis, so a revision of the anastomosis with thrombectomy was necessary.

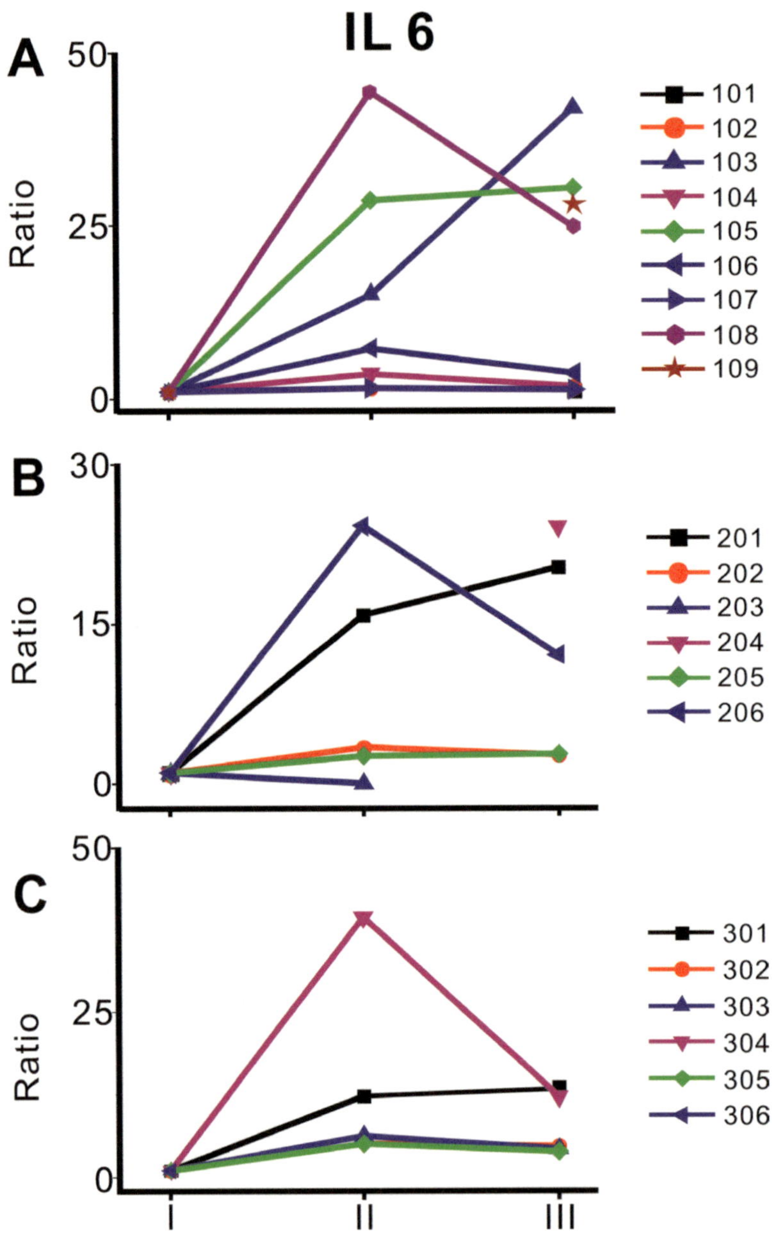

Figure 4. Line graphs of concentration ratios for IL6 from osteo-cutaneous flaps (A), muscle flaps (B), and skin flaps (C). Individual ratios were calculated from protein concentrations: I: artery/artery, II: Vein 1/artery, and III: Vein 2/artery. Patient IDs (**Table 1**) and respective symbols are shown at the right.

In sum, subgroup analysis confirmed that the dynamics of protein concentration differences of IL6 and IL8 correlated with I/R and seemed capable to characterize I/R-related processes on a molecular level for both the patients that showed clinical conspicuities or complications and those that did not. These concentration differences point toward a (transient) activation of leukocytes.

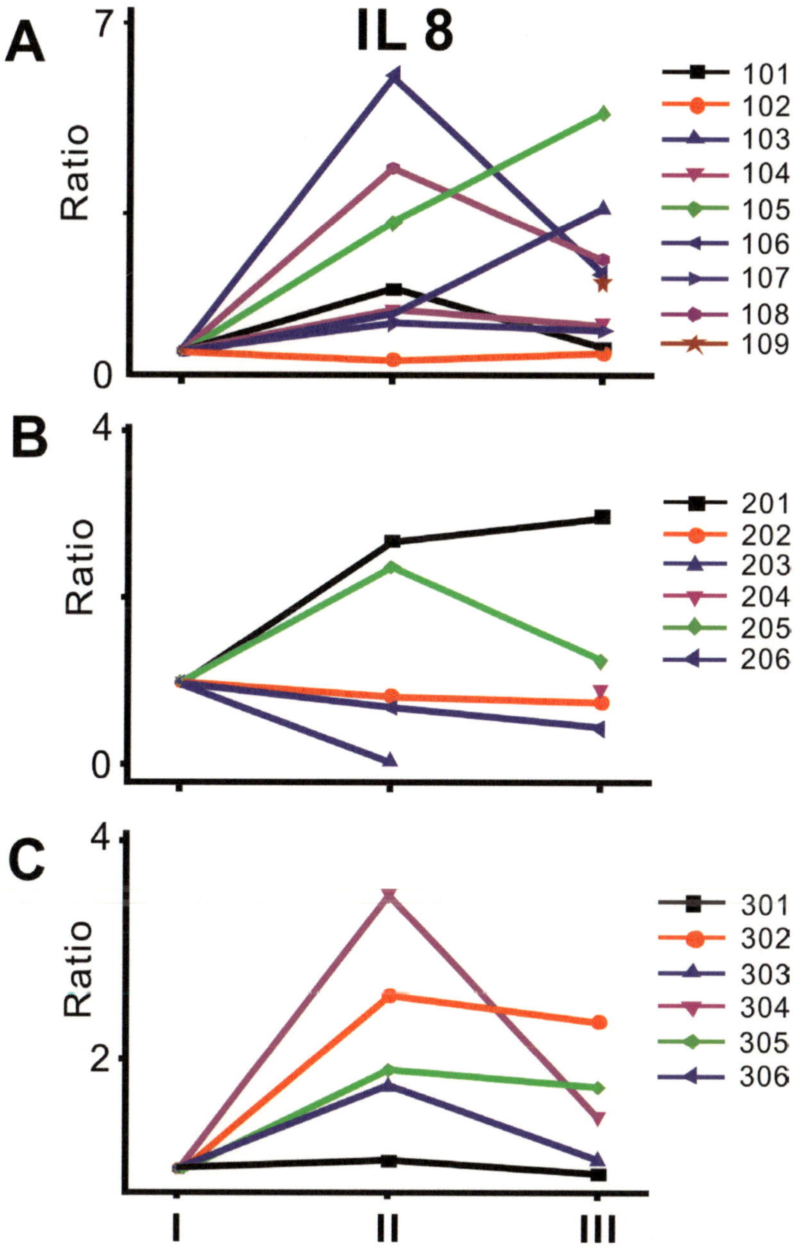

Figure 5. Line graphs of concentration ratios for IL8 from osteo-cutaneous flaps (A), muscle flaps (B), and skin flaps (C). Individual ratios were calculated from protein concentrations: I: artery/artery, II: Vein 1/artery, and III: Vein 2/artery. Patient IDs (**Table 1**) and respective symbols are shown at the right.

2.5. Conclusion

The dynamic nature of the circulating blood system and its constituents reflects diverse physiological or pathological states and, together with the ease with which blood can be sampled, makes it a logical choice for biomarker investigations [28]. Based on the inspection of the individual protein profiles of 18 cytokines and growth factors in the investigated study cohort (**Table 3**), IL8 and IL6 showed dynamic changes within the measured time frame.

IL6 together with TNFα and IL1β belongs to the so-called pro-inflammatory cytokines. IL6 is supposed to activate the coagulation system in experimental models, due to cross-links

Classification[a]	**Cytokine/growth factor**	**Protein family**	**Receptor**[b,c]	**Cytokine/growth factor target cell types**[c,d]
Dynamic change[e]	IL8	Cytokine/chemokine	CXCR1, E482	Neutrophils, basophils, CD8 T cells, epithelial and endothelial cells
	IL6	Cytokine/interleukin	CD126, CD130	T cells, B cells
No dynamic change[f]	MCP1	Cytokine/chemokine	CCR2	T cell monocytes, NK cells, B cells, endothelial cells
	bFGF	Growth factor (fibroblast)	FGFR	Epithelial cells
	GRO	Cytokine/chemokine	CXCR2	Neutrophils, fibroblasts, melanoma cells
	Fractalkine	Cytokine/chemokine	CX3CR1	Activated T cells, neutrophils, NK cells
	GMCSF	Cytokine/interleukin	CD116, βc	Bone marrow progenitors
	IP 10	Cytokine/chemokine	CXCR3A, CXCR3B	Activated T cells, NK cells, B cells, endothelial cells
	TNF α	Cytokine (TNF)	CD120a, CD120b	T cells, B cells, endothelial cells
	MIP 1α	Cytokine/chemokine	CCR1, CCR5	Immune cells, smooth muscle cells, endothelial cells
	IL10	Cytokine/interleukin	IL-10Rα, IL-10Rβc	Macrophages, T cells
	VEGF	Growth factor (vascular endothelial)	VEGFR	Vascular endothelial cells, hematopoietic stem cells, megakaryocytes
	IFNγ	Cytokine/interleukin	CD119, IFNGR2	Monocytes, endothelial cells, macrophages

Classification[a]	Cytokine/growth factor	Protein family	Receptor[b,c]	Cytokine/growth factor target cell types[c,d]
Undetermined	sCD40L	Cytokine (TNF)	CD40	Dendritic cells, B cells, macrophages
	TGF α	Growth factor (EGF-like domain)	EGFR	Epithelial cells
	IL1β	Cytokine/interleukin	CD121a, CD121b	T cells, macrophages
	IL12P40	Cytokine/interleukin	IL-12β1c + IL-12β2	NK cells, T cells
	TNFβ	Cytokine (TNF)	CD120a, CD120b	T cells, macrophages

[a]Comparisons of means of protein concentrations between sampling time points artery, Vein 1, and Vein 2.
[b]Baggiolini et al. [29].
[c]Janeway et al. [30].
[d]Huret et al. [31].
[e]Means are different between sampling time points artery, Vein 1, and Vein 2.
[f]Means are similar between sampling time points artery, Vein 1, and Vein 2.

Table 3. Classification of proteins according to their averaged plasma concentrations.

between inflammation and coagulation [32, 33]. Activated coagulation can result in microvascular thrombosis that possibly increases I/R injury [34]. Myocardial ischemia studies assume that changes in coagulation affect the resolution of ischemia during reperfusion due to changes in no-flow regions [35, 36]. In mice, IL6 deficiency reduced myocardial infarct size at 3 h reperfusion from which it was concluded that IL6 contributed to the development of infarct size in the early phase of reperfusion [37]. These results correspond to significantly elevated concentrations of IL6 in the venous blood samples of patients that experienced long ischemia periods.

IL8 is a prototypical member of the CXC chemokine family. Chemokines control innate immune cell trafficking between the bone marrow, blood, and peripheral tissues during inflammation. IL8 is a potent chemoattractant for neutrophils in vitro [38]. It has been reported to be a chemoattractant for a subset of T-lymphocytes [39]. IL8 is also called neutrophil-activating protein 1 (NAP-1) because it stimulates release of neutrophil granules. Like many other chemoattractants, IL8 induces re-arrangement of the cytoskeleton, changes in intracellular Ca^{2+} levels, activation of integrins, exocytosis of granule proteins, and respiratory burst [40]. IL8 concentration dynamics results in the here described study are consistent with published data, demonstrating the potential of IL8 as a marker protein of I/R injury in transplantation surgery. Interestingly, in cases of clinical conspicuities or complications, IL6 and IL8 react differently as compared to inconspicuous cases.

The activated forms of both macrophages and keratinocytes can release a number of inflammatory and cytotoxic active molecules that play essential roles in wound repair and/or tissue damage [41–43]. Macrophages, by secreting IL6, were suggested to interact with keratinocytes which are associated with epithelialization [44]. IL8 has a profound effect on the migration of keratinocytes which is again critical to wound epithelialization [45]. In vitro experiments on the effect of recombinant human IL8 on keratinocyte proliferation revealed a rise in cell numbers, whereas in vivo topically applied IL8 on human skin grafts in a chimeric mouse model enhanced re-epithelialization due to elevated numbers of mitotic keratinocytes [46]. The dynamic occurrence of chemokines IL8, GROα, MCP-1, IP-10, and Mig in the different phases of wound healing was described in a skin repair model in adult humans [47].

3. Outlook

The concept of targeting receptor cells that bind to IL6 or IL8 might become of importance for clinical interventions with the aim to accelerate wound healing as well as to attenuate fibrosis in response to individually determined cytokine/growth factor concentrations (**Figure 6**). Sequential function of endogenous IL8 and IL6 in all phases of human wound healing suggests to administering appropriate medication [48] in case of overexpression.

For instance, the anti-interleukin-6 receptor monoclonal antibody, tocilizumab, which was approved for the treatment of inflammatory diseases [49], might be tested in an off-label clinical study for its effect in modulating immune responses during free flap healing. A similar therapeutic concept may make use of HuMab 10FB, a fully human mAb against IL8, which

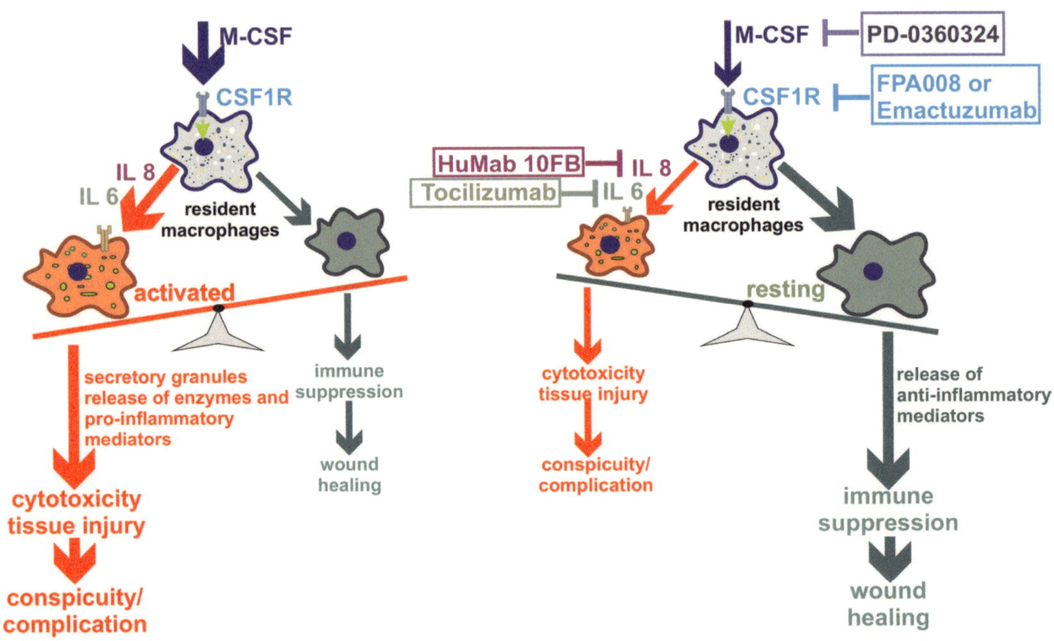

Figure 6. Implications of leucocytes (macrophages) in wound healing processes and clinical management without (left) and with (right) neutralizing antibody-based medication. Overproduced cytotoxic mediators or their receptors may be targeted. Pro-inflammatory mediators and enzymes may be clinically managed, whereas anti-inflammatory mediators would not be affected.

binds a discontinuous epitope on IL8 overlapping the receptor binding site, and it is capable to interrupt IL8 activity in vivo [50]. Both therapeutic antibodies would neutralize increased levels of interleukins and directly interfere in leukocyte signaling with potentially positive effects on tissue and wound healing processes.

These results indicate the sequential function of endogenous MCSF [51], IL8, and IL6 in wound healing which in case of overexpression may be clinically managed by administering appropriate medication, i.e., management of an individuals' systemic inflammatory status to reduce or even prevent conspicuities and complications during perioperative and postoperative periods. Concomitant medication may become an important if not indispensable part of state-of-the-art flap surgery in the future.

4. Appendix

4.1. Clinical specimen collection

Presented and discussed data are from a study that was approved by the Institutional Review Board of the University Hospital Zurich, Switzerland (StV 8-2009). Written informed consent was obtained from all participating patients. Three groups of free flap transfers were defined: (i) muscle flaps, e.g., gracilis flap, latissimus dorsi flap, serratus anterior flap, (ii) fascio-cutaneous flaps, e.g., radialis flap, anterolateral thigh flap, and (iii) osteo-cutaneous flaps, i.e., fibula flaps. Clinical measurements include the ischemia time, flap weight, length of bone (in fibula flaps), and the dimension of the skin island. Patients qualified for the study had to be with normal weight (BMI 20–25), non-diabetics, in no manifest infection situation, and of good health with no essential diseases besides the main diagnosis (**Table 1**). Blood samples were taken intraoperatively prior to arterial anastomosis from the arterial inflow and after arterial anastomosis from the venous flap outflow. Vein 1 samples were taken directly after anastomosis and Vein 2 samples 2 min after collecting Vein 1 samples in 1.5 mL portions using S-Monovette® Lithium Heparin syringes (Monovette®, Sarstedt, Germany). Blood samples were immediately subjected to sedimentation of blood cells by centrifugation at 2000 g at room temperature for 15 min. Plasma was aspirated and sterile-filtered (0.2 μm pore size) [52]. Five samples had to be excluded from the study because of too less material after centrifugation and sterile filtration: patient 109 (Vein 1), patient 203 (Vein 2), patient 204 (Vein 1), and patient 306 (Vein 1 and Vein 2). In total, 58 plasma samples had been collected. Aliquots of 100 μL per portion were stored at −80°C prior to further analysis.

4.2. Multiplexed bead-based immunoassay

The Human Cytokine/Chemokine Magnetic Bead Panel from Milliplex® (Map kit HCYTOMAG-60K, Billerica, MA, USA) contained antibodies against 18 proteins that were delivered immobilized onto color-coded beads. All kit reagents were brought to 25°C. Then, the two quality control samples were reconstituted with 250 μL deionized water, each. Serum matrix was reconstituted with 1.0 mL deionized water. The human cytokine standard mixture was reconstituted with 250 μL deionized water to give a 10,000 pg/mL concentration for each of the standards. This solution was serially diluted by a factor of 5 and yielded in diluted human cytokine standards with the following concentrations: 10,000, 2000, 400, 80, 16, and 3.2 pg/mL. Next, each antibody-bead containing vial was sonicated for 30 s and then vortexed for 1 min. Sixty microliters of antibody-bead slurry from each of the 18 vials was added to the mixing bottle, and 1.92 mL "bead diluent" was added to achieve a final volume of 3.0 mL. Two 96-well plates were pre-wetted with 200 μL wash buffer, each. After sealing, the plates were fixed on the shaker (Heidolph® Promax 2020, Schwabach, Germany) and gently agitated for 10 min at room temperature. The wash buffer was decanted, and the residual amount was removed by inverting the plates and gently tapping onto absorbent towels for several times. Twenty-five microliters, each, of all six diluted human cytokine standards and the two quality control samples were added into their dedicated wells. Twenty-five microliters, each, of assay buffer were added to two "background" wells and to the wells that were dedicated to patient samples. Second, 25 μL of serum matrix was added into each of the diluted human cytokine standard wells, the background wells, and the quality control sample wells. Twenty-five microliters of each patient plasma was added into one of the patient sample wells. Twenty-five microliters, each, of antibody-bead slurry from the mixing bottle was added to all the wells. Afterwards, plates were sealed and incubated in the dark for 18 h at 4°C on the plate shaker. Solvents from each well were removed, avoiding loss of beads, and beads were washed twice with wash buffer (200 μL, for each well, 1 min incubation). After removal of wash buffer, 25 μL, each, of detection antibody solution was added to all wells. After 1 h incubation at 25°C, 25 μL of phycoerythrin-loaded streptavidin containing solution was added to all wells. The plates were sealed again, covered with aluminum foil, and then fixed on the plate shaker for 30 min at 25°C. Subsequently, beads were washed twice with wash buffer (200 μL, for each well, 1 min incubation). After removal of wash buffer, 150 μL of sheath fluid (Bio-Rad Laboratories, Hercules, CA, USA) was added to all wells and beads were resuspended on the plate shaker for 5 min. Plates were placed into the Bio-Plex suspension array 200 System (Bio-Rad Laboratories, Hercules, CA, USA), which had been calibrated with Bio-Plex® 200 calibration kit and validated with Bio-Plex® validation kit 4.0 (Bio-Rad Laboratories, Hercules, CA, USA). Measurement settings were as follows: data acquisition, 50 beads per region; sample size, 100 μL; and doublet discriminator gate, 5000–25,000 (low photomultiplier tube). The Bio-Plex suspension array 200 reader system contains a red laser for identification of the bead which is analyzed and a green laser for quantification of fluorescence intensity of phycoerythrin-loaded streptavidin. All standards, controls, background, and plasma samples were prepared in duplicate and measured once. From the 2088 independent measurements, the Bio-Plex® manager 6.1 software (Bio-Rad Laboratories, Hercules, CA, USA) calculated median fluorescence intensity (MFI) and standard deviations of each duplicate recording. Fluorescence values of human cytokine standards were plotted as standard curves which were used for determining plasma concentrations (pg/mL) based on their fluorescence intensities of all proteins and all time points. In total, 1044 data points (raw data set) were stored as Excel files.

4.3. Full analysis set and per protocol set

Data from the raw data set were inspected for completeness and categorized into three groups based on the detection rates. Group I contained those cytokines and growth factors (CGFs) for which plasma protein concentrations could be determined in over 80% of all samples. Group

II included those CGFs for which plasma protein concentrations could be determined in over 60% but less than 80% of all samples. Group III contained proteins whose concentrations were determined in less than 60% of all samples and sCD40L which did not pass the QC test. In both, group I and group II proteins, the missing values were imputed using the lower limit of quantitation (LLOQ) except for MCP1 for which upper limit of quantitation (ULOQ) was imputed. After imputing, the "full analysis set (FAS)" contained a total of 1044 curated data points (data not shown). The "per protocol set (PPS)" was generated out of the "full analysis set (FAS)" by including only group I and group II CGFs, resulting in 754 data points.

4.4. Biostatistical analysis

Statistical analyses were performed using the PPS with the IBM statistics software SPSS (version 20.0, SPSS Inc., Chicago, USA). Linear fit analysis between ischemia time and protein concentration was performed using the Origin statistics software (version. 8.1 G; OriginLab Corporation, Northampton, MA, USA). Linear regression was performed to calculate R^2 values, and ANOVA tests were performed to calculate p values to estimate whether protein concentration was related to the ischemia time [53]. Hierarchical cluster analysis and dendrogram presentation were performed on the Knowledge Discovery Environment (KDE) platform (InforSense Ltd., London, UK). Parameter settings were single linkage and Euclidean distance. CV% for each analyte was calculated as the ratio of the standard deviation to the plasma mean concentration [25, 26].

Author details

Juliane C. Finke[1,2#], Jingzhi Yang[1#], Marius Bredell[3], Uwe von Fritschen[2] and Michael O. Glocker[1*]

*Address all correspondence to: michael.glocker@uni-rostock.de

1 Proteome Center Rostock, University Medicine and Natural Science Faculty, University of Rostock, Rostock, Germany

2 Division of Plastic Surgery and Hand Surgery, HELIOS Clinic Emil von Behring, Berlin, Germany

3 Department of Cranio-Maxillofacial and Oral Surgery, University Hospital of Zürich, Zürich, Switzerland

# These authors contributed equally.

References

[1] Bui DT, Cordeiro PG, Hu QY, Disa JJ, Pusic A, Mehrara BJ. Free flap reexploration: Indications, treatment, and outcomes in 1193 free flaps. Plastic and Reconstructive Surgery. 2007;**119**(7):2092-2100. DOI: 10.1097/01.prs.0000260598.24376.e1

[2] Eisenhardt SU, Schmidt Y, Karaxha G, Iblher N, Penna V, Torio-Padron N, Stark GB, Bannasch H. Monitoring molecular changes induced by ischemia/reperfusion in human free muscle flap tissue samples. Annals of Plastic Surgery. 2012;**68**(2):202-208. DOI: 10.1097/SAP.0b013e3181f77ba5

[3] Cerra FB, Lajos TZ, Montes M, Siegel JH. Hemorrhagic infarction: A reperfusion injury following prolonged myocardial ischemic anoxia. Surgery. 1975;**78**(1):95-104

[4] Khalil AA, Aziz FA, Hall JC. Reperfusion injury. Plastic and Reconstructive Surgery. 2006;**117**(3):1024-1033. DOI: 10.1097/01.prs.0000204766.17127.54

[5] [5] Baumeister S, Ofer N, Kleist C, Terne P, Opelz G, Gebhard MM, Germann G, Heitmann C. Reduction of skeletal muscle injury in composite tissue allotransplantation by heat stress preconditioning. Plastic and Reconstructive Surgery. 2004;**114**(7):1832-1841

[6] [6] Eming SA, Hammerschmidt M, Krieg T, Roers A. Interrelation of immunity and tissue repair or regeneration. Seminars in Cell and Developmental Biology. 2009;**20**(5):517-527. DOI: 10.1016/j.semcdb.2009.04.009

[7] Jennings RB, Murry CE, Steenbergen C Jr, Reimer KA. Development of cell injury in sustained acute ischemia. Circulation. 1990;**82**(3 Suppl):II2-12

[8] Nolte D, Lehr HA, Messmer K. Adenosine inhibits postischemic leukocyte-endothelium interaction in postcapillary venules of the hamster. American Journal of Physiology. 1991;**261**(3 Pt 2):H651-655

[9] Farhood A, McGuire GM, Manning AM, Miyasaka M, Smith CW, Jaeschke H. Intercellular adhesion molecule 1 (ICAM-1) expression and its role in neutrophil-induced ischemia-reperfusion injury in rat liver. Journal of Leukocyte Biology. 1995;**57**(3):368-374

[10] Rashid MA, William-Olsson G. Are leukocytosis and lipid peroxidation involved in ischemic or reperfusion injury in cardiac surgery? Thoracic and Cardiovascular Surgeon. 1991;**39**(4):193-195. DOI: 10.1055/s-2007-1022707

[11] Zimmerman BJ, Granger DN. Mechanisms of reperfusion injury. American Journal of the Medical Sciences. 1994;**307**(4):284-292

[12] Lazarus B, Messina A, Barker JE, Hurley JV, Romeo R, Morrison WA, Knight KR. The role of mast cells in ischaemia-reperfusion injury in murine skeletal muscle. Journal of Pathology. 2000;**191**(4):443-448. DOI: 10.1002/1096-9896(2000)9999:9999<::AID-PATH666>3.0.CO;2-L

[13] Schmidt Y, Bannasch H, Eisenhardt SU. Ischemia-reperfusion injury leads to significant tissue damage in free flap surgery. Plastic and Reconstructive Surgery. 2012;**129**(1):174e-175e;author reply 175e-176e. DOI: 10.1097/PRS.0b013e3182362e53

[14] Wang Y, Yamamoto Y, Kuninaka Y, Kondo T, Furukawa F. Forensic potential of MMPs and CC chemokines for wound age determination. Journal of the Forensic Science. 2015;**60**(6):1511-1515. DOI: 10.1111/1556-4029.12831

[15] Chen ZG, Persons B, Lin L, Lineaweaver WC, Zhang F. Vascular endothelial growth factor upregulates inducible nitric oxide synthase expression in the muscle flap ischemia model

in the rat. Journal of Reconstructive Microsurgery. 2009;**25**(4):219-225. DOI: 10.1055/s-0028-1104550

[16] Dragu A, Schnurer S, Surmann-Schmitt C, von der Mark K, Sturzl M, Unglaub F, Wolf MB, Leffler M, Beier JP, Kneser U, Horch RE. Gene expression analysis of ischaemia and reperfusion in human microsurgical free muscle tissue transfer. Journal of Cellular and Molecular Medicine. 2011;**15**(4):983-993. DOI: 10.1111/j.1582-4934.2010.01061.x

[17] Leng SX, McElhaney JE, Walston JD, Xie D, Fedarko NS, Kuchel GA. ELISA and multiplex technologies for cytokine measurement in inflammation and aging research. The Journals of Gerontology. Series A: Biological Sciences and Medical Sciences. The Journals of Gerontology. Series A: Biological Sciences and Medical Sciences. 2008;**63**(8):879-884

[18] Vaucher J, Marques-Vidal P, Waeber G, Vollenweider P. Cytokines and hs-CRP levels in individuals treated with low-dose aspirin for cardiovascular prevention: A population-based study (CoLaus Study). Cytokine. 2014;**66**(2):95-100. DOI: 10.1016/j.cyto.2014.01.003

[19] Yurkovetsky ZR, Kirkwood JM, Edington HD, Marrangoni AM, Velikokhatnaya L, Winans MT, Gorelik E, Lokshin AE. Multiplex analysis of serum cytokines in melanoma patients treated with interferon-alpha2b. Clinical Cancer Research. 2007;**13**(8):2422-2428. DOI: 10.1158/1078-0432.CCR-06-1805

[20] Geyer AI, Kraus T, Roberts T, Wisnivesky J, Eber CD, Hiensch R, Moran TM. Plasma level of interferon gamma induced protein 10 is a marker of sarcoidosis disease activity. Cytokine. 2013;**64**(1):152-157. DOI: 10.1016/j.cyto.2013.07.010

[21] Damas JK, Boullier A, Waehre T, Smith C, Sandberg WJ, Green S, Aukrust P, Quehenberger O. Expression of fractalkine (CX3CL1) and its receptor, CX3CR1, is elevated in coronary artery disease and is reduced during statin therapy. Arteriosclerosis Thrombosis and Vascular Biology. 2005;**25**(12):2567-2572. DOI: 10.1161/01.ATV.0000190672.36490.7b

[22] Hang H, Yuan S, Yang Q, Yuan D, Liu Q. Multiplex bead array assay of plasma cytokines in type 2 diabetes mellitus with diabetic retinopathy. Molecular Vision. 2014;**20**:1137-1145

[23] Lee J, Kim Y, Lim J, Kim M, Han K. G-CSF and GM-CSF concentrations and receptor expression in peripheral blood leukemic cells from patients with chronic myelogenous leukemia. Annals of Clinical and Laboratory Science. 2008;**38**(4):331-337

[24] Larsson A, Skoldenberg E, Ericson H. Serum and plasma levels of FGF-2 and VEGF in healthy blood donors. Angiogenesis. 2002;**5**(1-2):107-110

[25] O'Connell MA, Belanger BA, Haaland PD. Calibration and assay development using the four-parameter logistic model. Chemometrics and Intelligent Laboratory Systems. 1993;**20**:97-114

[26] Quinn CP, Semenova VA, Elie CM, Romero-Steiner S, Greene C, Li H, Stamey K, Steward-Clark E, Schmidt DS, Mothershed E, Pruckler J, Schwartz S, Benson RF, Helsel LO, Holder PF, Johnson SE, Kellum M, Messmer T, Thacker WL, Besser L, Plikaytis BD, Taylor TH Jr, Freeman AE, Wallace KJ, Dull P, Sejvar J, Bruce E, Moreno R, Schuchat A, Lingappa JR, Martin SK, Walls J, Bronsdon M, Carlone GM, Bajani-Ari M, Ashford DA,

Stephens DS, Perkins BA. Specific, sensitive, and quantitative enzyme-linked immunosorbent assay for human immunoglobulin G antibodies to anthrax toxin protective antigen. Emerging Infectious Diseases. 2002;**8**(10):1103-1110. DOI: 10.3201/eid0810.020380

[27] Staples E, Ingram RJ, Atherton JC, Robinson K. Optimising the quantification of cytokines present at low concentrations in small human mucosal tissue samples using Luminex assays. Journal of Immunological Methods. 2013;**394**(1-2):1-9. DOI: 10.1016/j.jim.2013.04.009

[28] Hanash SM, Pitteri SJ, Faca VM. Mining the plasma proteome for cancer biomarkers. Nature. 2008;**452**(7187):571-579. DOI:10.1038/nature06916

[29] Baggiolini M, Loetscher P. Chemokines in inflammation and immunity. Immunology Today. 2000;**21**(9):418-420

[30] Janeway C, Paul Travers J, Walport M, Shlomchik M. Immunobiology: The Immune System in Health and Disease. New York: Garland Science; 2001

[31] Huret JL, Ahmad M, Arsaban M, Bernheim A, Cigna J, Desangles F, Guignard JC, Jacquemot-Perbal MC, Labarussias M, Leberre V, Malo A, Morel-Pair C, Mossafa H, Potier JC, Texier G, Viguie F, Yau Chun Wan-Senon S, Zasadzinski A, Dessen P. Atlas of genetics and cytogenetics in oncology and haematology in 2013. Nucleic Acids Research. 2013;**41**(Database issue):D920-924. DOI: 10.1093/nar/gks1082

[32] van der Poll T, Levi M, Hack CE, ten Cate H, van Deventer SJ, Eerenberg AJ, de Groot ER, Jansen J, Gallati H, Buller HR, et al. Elimination of interleukin 6 attenuates coagulation activation in experimental endotoxemia in chimpanzees. Journal of Experimental Medicine. 1994;**179**(4):1253-1259

[33] Stouthard JM, Levi M, Hack CE, Veenhof CH, Romijn HA, Sauerwein HP, van der Poll T. Interleukin-6 stimulates coagulation, not fibrinolysis, in humans. Thrombosis and Haemostasis. 1996;**76**(5):738-742

[34] Erlich JH, Boyle EM, Labriola J, Kovacich JC, Santucci RA, Fearns C, Morgan EN, Yun W, Luther T, Kojikawa O, Martin TR, Pohlman TH, Verrier ED, Mackman N. Inhibition of the tissue factor-thrombin pathway limits infarct size after myocardial ischemia-reperfusion injury by reducing inflammation. American Journal of Pathology. 2000;**157**(6):1849-1862. DOI: 10.1016/S0002-9440(10)64824-9

[35] Li RA, Leppo M, Miki T, Seino S, Marban E. Molecular basis of electrocardiographic ST-segment elevation. Circulation Research. 2000;**87**(10):837-839

[36] Gehrmann J, Frantz S, Maguire CT, Vargas M, Ducharme A, Wakimoto H, Lee RT, Berul CI. Electrophysiological characterization of murine myocardial ischemia and infarction. Basic Research in Cardiology. 2001;**96**(3):237-250

[37] Jong WM, ten Cate H, Linnenbank AC, de Boer OJ, Reitsma PH, de Winter RJ, Zuurbier CJ. Reduced acute myocardial ischemia-reperfusion injury in IL-6-deficient mice employing a closed-chest model. Inflammation Research. 2016. DOI: 10.1007/s00011-016-0931-4

[38] Palomino DC, Marti LC. Chemokines and immunity. Einstein (Sao Paulo). 2015;**13**(3):469-473. DOI: 10.1590/S1679-45082015RB3438

[39] Huber AR, Kunkel SL, Todd RF 3rd, Weiss SJ. Regulation of transendothelial neutrophil migration by endogenous interleukin-8. Science. 1991;**254**(5028):99-102

[40] Paccaud JP, Schifferli JA, Baggiolini M. NAP-1/IL-8 induces up-regulation of CR1 receptors in human neutrophil leukocytes. Biochemical and Biophysical Research Communications. 1990;**166**(1):187-192

[41] Raja, Sivamani K, Garcia MS, Isseroff RR. Wound re-epithelialization: Modulating keratinocyte migration in wound healing. Frontiers in Bioscience. 2007;**12**:2849-2868

[42] Laskin DL, Sunil VR, Gardner CR, Laskin JD. Macrophages and tissue injury: Agents of defense or destruction? Annual Review of Pharmacology and Toxicology. 2011;**51**:267-288. DOI: 10.1146/annurev.pharmtox.010909.105812

[43] Koh TJ, DiPietro LA. Inflammation and wound healing: the role of the macrophage. Expert Reviews in Molecular Medicine. 2011;**13**:e23. DOI: 10.1017/S1462399411001943

[44] Rodero MP, Khosrotehrani K. Skin wound healing modulation by macrophages. International Journal of Clinical and Experimental Pathology. 2010;**3**(7):643-653

[45] Jiang WG, Sanders AJ, Ruge F, Harding KG. Influence of interleukin-8 (IL-8) and IL-8 receptors on the migration of human keratinocytes, the role of PLC-gamma and potential clinical implications. Experimental and Therapeutic Medicine. 2012;**3**(2):231-236. DOI: 10.3892/etm.2011.402

[46] Rennekampff HO, Hansbrough JF, Kiessig V, Dore C, Sticherling M, Schroder JM. Bioactive interleukin-8 is expressed in wounds and enhances wound healing. Journal of Surgical Research. 2000;**93**(1):41-54. DOI: 10.1006/jsre.2000.5892

[47] Engelhardt E, Toksoy A, Goebeler M, Debus S, Brocker EB, Gillitzer R. Chemokines IL-8, GROalpha, MCP-1, IP-10, and Mig are sequentially and differentially expressed during phase-specific infiltration of leukocyte subsets in human wound healing. American Journal of Pathology. 1998;**153**(6):1849-1860

[48] Maude SL, Teachey DT, Porter DL, Grupp SA. CD19-targeted chimeric antigen receptor T-cell therapy for acute lymphoblastic leukemia. Blood. 2015;**125**(26):4017-4023. DOI: 10.1182/blood-2014-12-580068

[49] Scheller J, Chalaris A, Schmidt-Arras D, Rose-John S. The pro- and anti-inflammatory properties of the cytokine interleukin-6. Biochimica et Biophysica Acta. 2011;**1813**(5):878-888. DOI: 10.1016/j.bbamcr.2011.01.034

[50] Skov L, Beurskens FJ, Zachariae CO, Reitamo S, Teeling J, Satijn D, Knudsen KM, Boot EP, Hudson D, Baadsgaard O, Parren PW, van de Winkel JG. IL-8 as antibody therapeutic target in inflammatory diseases: Reduction of clinical activity in palmoplantar pustulosis. Journal of Immunology. 2008;**181**(1):669-679

[51] Yang J, Finke JC, Yang J, Percy AJ, von Fritschen U, Borchers CH, Glocker MO. Early risk prognosis of free-flap transplant failure by quantitation of the macrophage colony-stimulating factor in patient plasma using 2-dimensional liquid-chromatography multiple reaction monitoring-mass spectrometry. Medicine. 2016;**95**(39):e4808. DOI: 10.1097/MD.0000000000004808

[52] Koy C, Heitner JC, Woisch R, Kreutzer M, Serrano-Fernandez P, Gohlke R, Reimer T, Glocker MO. Cryodetector mass spectrometry profiling of plasma samples for HELLP diagnosis: An exploratory study. Proteomics. 2005;**5**(12):3079-3087. DOI: 10.1002/pmic.200402098

[53] Montgomery DC. In: Anderson W, editor. Design and Analysis of Experiments. United States of America: John Wiley & Sons; 2001. pp. 65-75

Chapter 2

Experimental Rat Flap Models

Merdan Serin and Mehmet Bayramicli

Additional information is available at the end of the chapter

http://dx.doi.org/10.5772/intechopen.69923

Abstract

Experimental flap surgery aims to increase our understanding of flap physiology and to test new surgical techniques to increase flap viability. Many experimental flap models have been described with the advancement of flap surgery and research. Most commonly used experimental flaps used in rats, including dorsal skin, flank, epigastric, oblique groin, pectoral, latissimus dorsi, rectus abdominis and fibula flaps, will be described.

Keywords: experimental flaps, rat, flap physiology

1. Introduction

Animal experiments performed on rats have played a crucial role in the development of flap surgery over the past years. There are many experimental rat flap surgery models. Main purposes of these models include understanding flap physiology, as a training tool for residents and to test new surgical techniques. The effect of pharmacological agents, delay procedures and different anastomosis techniques on flap survival can be studied on these models. The evaluation of the results of these experiments usually involves flap necrosis area calculation based on calibrated photographs, histological evaluation and angiographic imaging.

2. Skin flaps

2.1. Dorsal skin flap

This flap was described by McFarlane et al. [1] in 1965. This is one of the most commonly used flaps for random flap studies. This flap is raised based on a caudal pedicle from the dorsal rat skin. This flap was originally described as being 10×4 cm in dimension or as having a length-to-width ratio of 2,5/1. Later, this original description was modified to 9×3 and 10×3 dimensions, a modification that proved to demonstrate more consistent results [2]. Various flap viability ratios have been reported depending on dimension. The author believes that 9×3 cm flap provides the most consistent flap viability ratio (**Figure 1**).

Templates are commonly used to mark flap dimension on the skin before the flap elevation. It is important to note that these templates might result in inaccuracies due to the curvature of animal's body.

2.2. Flank flap

Syed et al. [3] described this flap as the skin area supplied by the iliac branch of iliolumbar artery. Its borders were from the back of 12th rib to the proximal part of the tail medially and the axillary line laterally. It was suggested as a consistent model for experimental flap research (**Figure 2**).

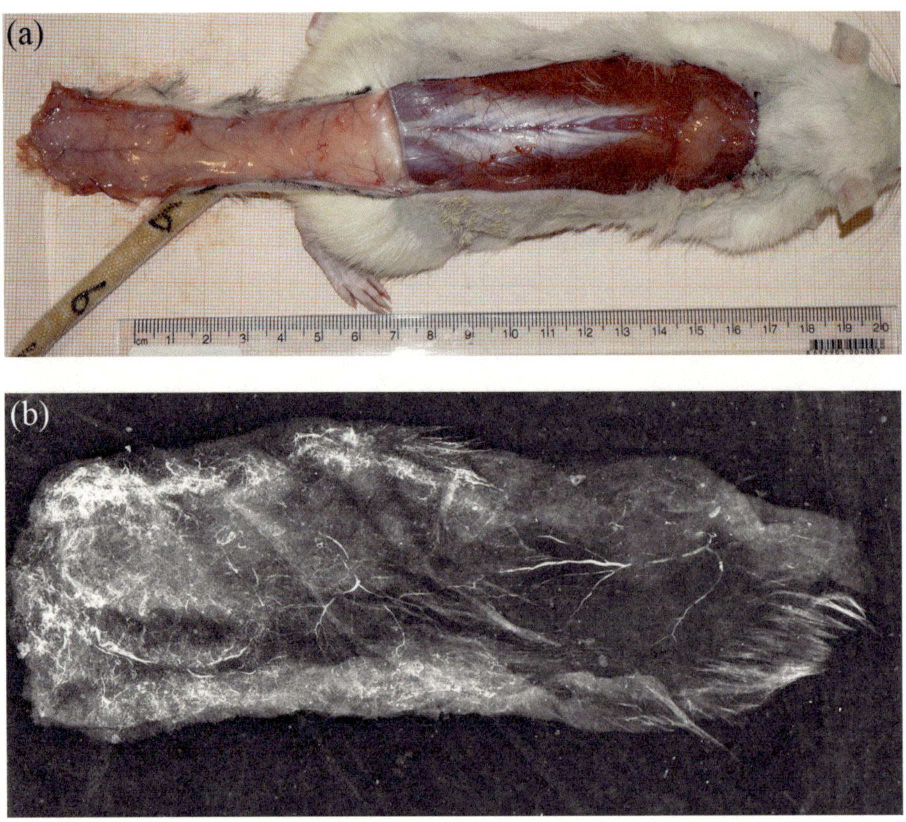

Figure 1. Dorsal skin flap. (A) Flap elevation and (B) angiographic image.

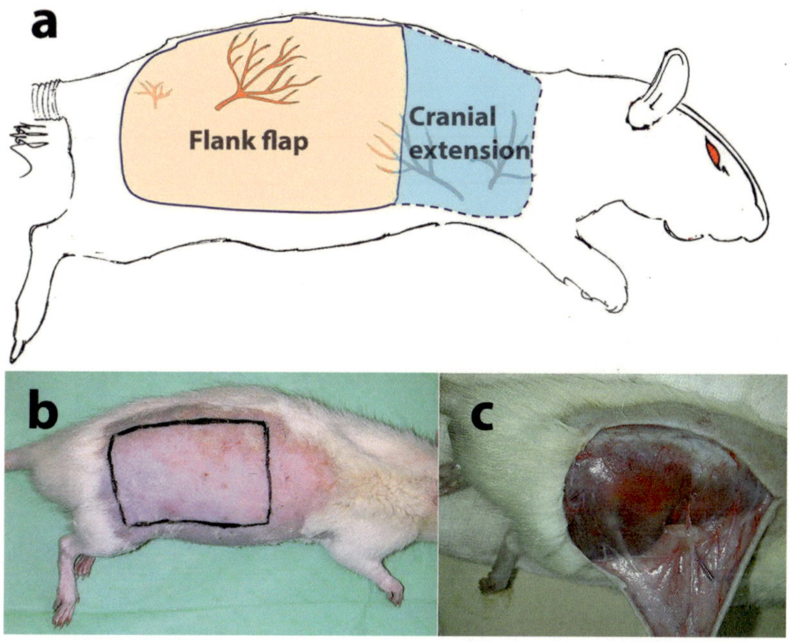

Figure 2. Flank flap. (a) Flank flap and its cranial extension; (b) skin marking and (c) flap elevation.

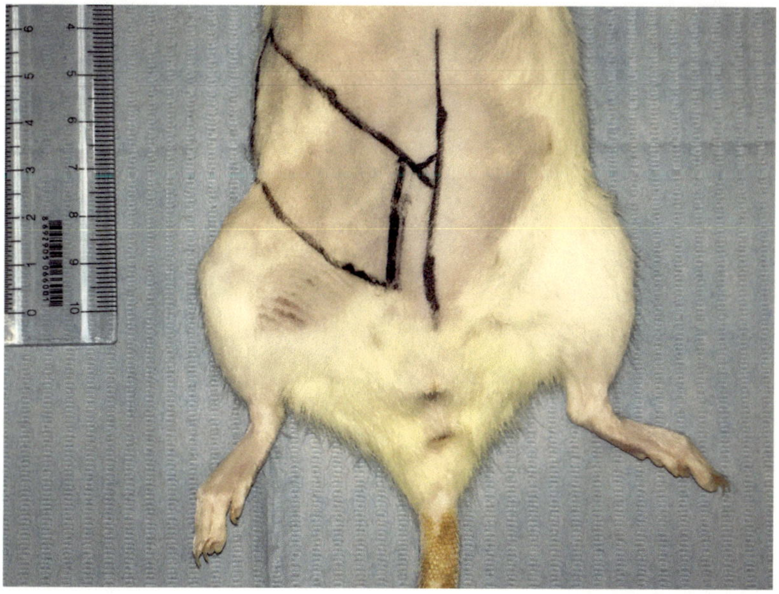

Figure 3. Oblique rat groin flap.

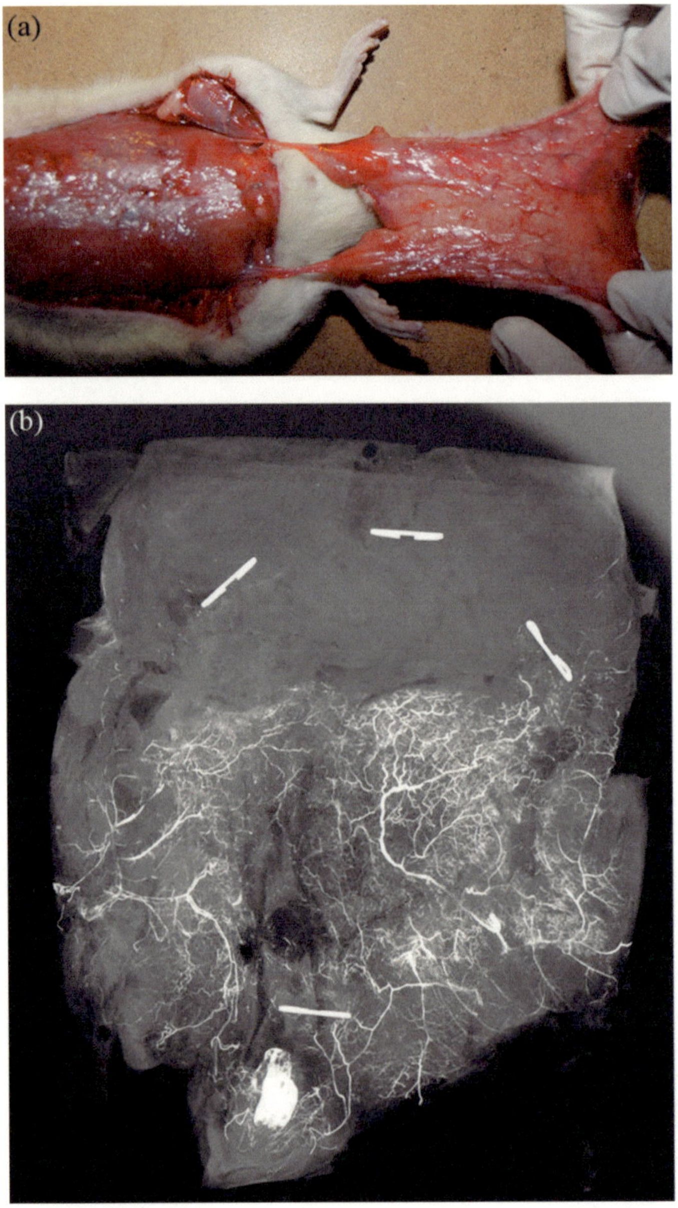

Figure 4. Epigastric flap. (A) Flap elevation and (B) angiographic image.

2.3. Epigastric flap

Finseth and Cutting [4] first described this flap back in 1978 as a neurovascular island flap. This flap is commonly used for axial flap studies and microvascular anastomosis studies. This flap is also commonly used in conjunction with angiographic studies. The flap is designed on superficial epigastric vessels which originate from the femoral artery. The superficial epigastric trunk divides into lateral and medial branches. The lateral branches have been reported to

http://dx.doi.org/10.5772/intechopen.69923

be variable by some studies [5]. The median vessels collateralize with the branches of internal mammary vessels. The lateral branches collateralize with lateral thoracic artery (**Figure 3**).

2.4. Oblique rat groin flap

Nishikawa et al. [6] described this flap in 1991. The purpose of this flap is to prevent flap neovascularization from its underlying bed, which could interfere with the results in certain type of studies. This flap is designed over adipose fat pads which act as a barrier for new vessel formation (**Figure 4**).

3. Muscle flaps

Various muscle flaps have been identified for research in rats. Other than those included in this section, adductor muscle flap [7], gracilis flap [8], gluteus maximus [9], gastrocnemius [10, 11], quadriceps femoris flap [12] and cremaster flaps have been described [13].

3.1. Pectoral flap

This flap was first defined by Zhang et al. [14]. It consists of two parts, superficial and profundus. These parts are supplied by separate neural and vascular systems. The profundus

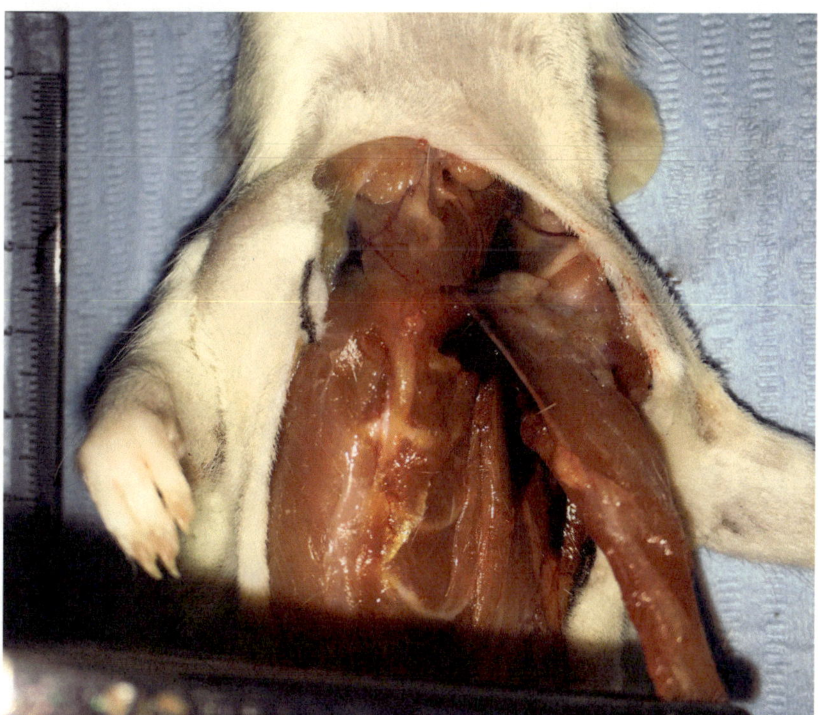

Figure 5. Pectoral flap.

part is in association with axillary vessels and is more commonly used for experimental studies (**Figure 5**).

3.2. Latissimus dorsi flap

Tilgner et al. [15] described the latissimus dorsi flap in rats. Rat latissimus dorsi muscle has a similar vascular anatomy when compared to humans. It is supplied by the thoracodorsal pedicle and five to six intercostal perforators. It is a suitable model for vascular delay studies and has been reported to have a consistent necrosis pattern [16] (**Figure 6**).

3.3. Rectus abdominis flap

This flap was described by Zhang et al. [17]. Myocutaneous flaps can be raised with this model. The skin island is designed over the anterior sheath of the rectus muscle. Inferior edge of the flap is planned 2.5 cm above the symphysis. The muscle is supplied by superior and inferior epigastric arteries and veins. Microvascular flap transplantation is possible with this model with average vessel diameter of 0.5 mm (**Figure 7**).

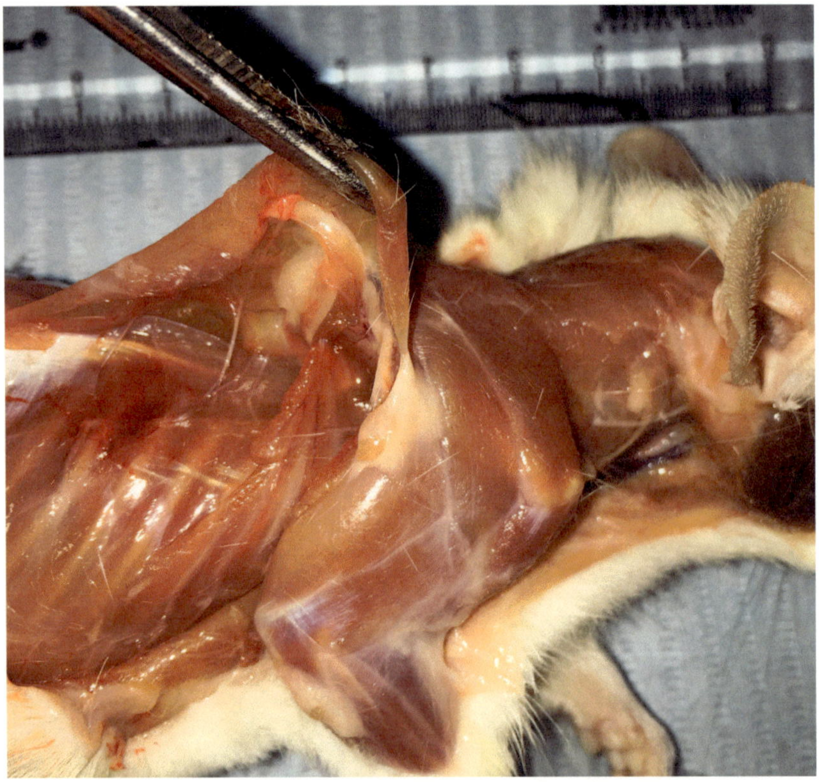

Figure 6. Latissimus dorsi muscle flap.

http://dx.doi.org/10.5772/intechopen.69923

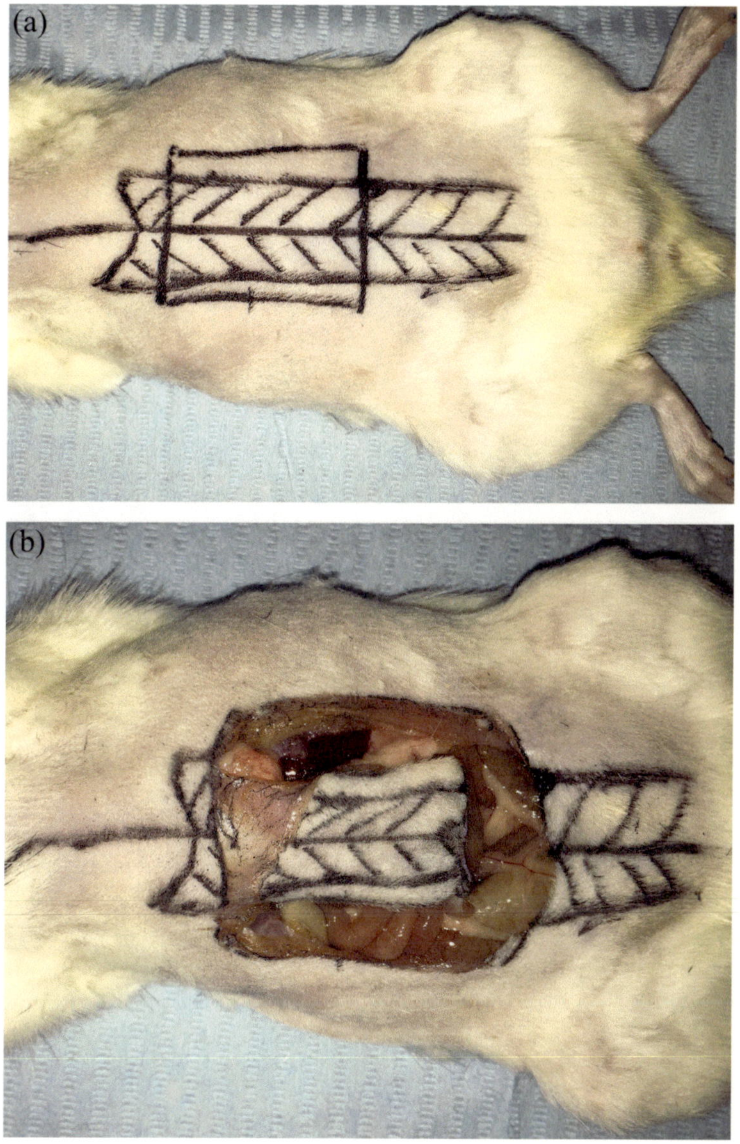

Figure 7. Rectus abdominis flap. (a) Flap design and (b) flap elevation.

4. Fibula flap

Fibula flap is one of the most common flaps used in mandibular reconstruction in clinical practice. Chen et al. [18] described the rat fibula bone flap as a free vascularized bone flap model. The flap is usually raised with a medial incision as opposed to humans in which a lateral approach is used. Flexor halluces muscle is usually included in the flap. Peroneal vessels that supply the flap originate from the popliteal and anterior tibial artery vessels (**Figure 8**).

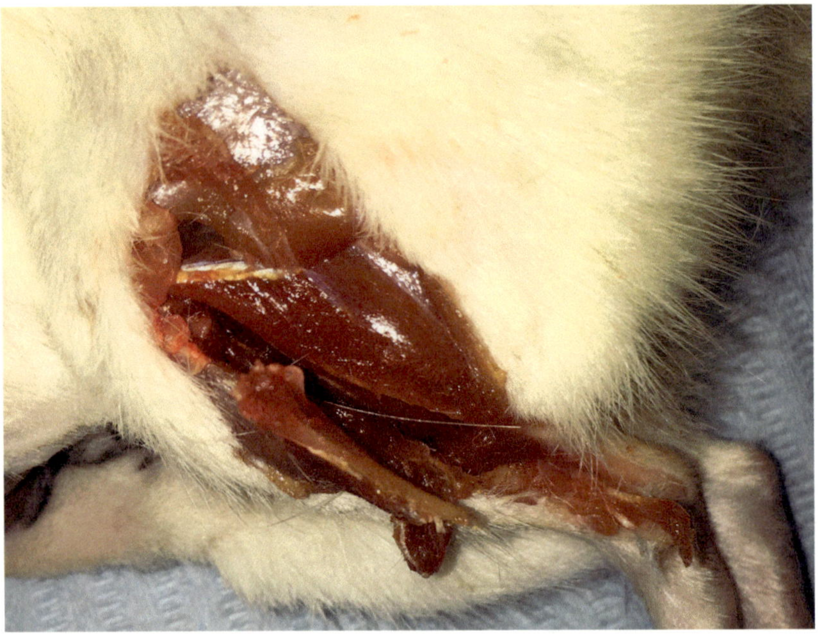

Figure 8. Fibula flap.

5. Conclusion

Rat models have been proven to be a very valuable tool for flap research. In spite of the developments in the field of cell cultures, in vitro studies are usually not as valuable as animal studies in this field. Although other animal models have been proposed, rats are by far the most commonly used species for these purposes. They are easier to maintain and more readily available. Although much more valuable than in vitro studies, rat experiments do also have their limitations. The application of the results of rat model experiments on human subjects may not always be possible. Differences in the life span and the wound healing processes between humans and rats should be considered.

Author details

Merdan Serin[1]* and Mehmet Bayramicli[2]

*Address all correspondence to: merdanserin@gmail.com

1 Plastic Surgery Clinic, Istanbul Training and Research Hospital, Turkey

2 Plastic Surgery Department, Marmara University Medical School, Turkey

References

[1] McFarlane RM, Deyoung G, Henry RA. The design of a pedicle flap in the rat to study necrosis and its prevention. Plastic and Reconstructive Surgery. 1965;**35**:177-182

[2] Kelly CP, et al. *A* new design of a dorsal flap in the rat to study skin necrosis and its prevention. Journal of Plastic, Reconstructive and Aesthetic Surgery. 2010;**63**(9): 1553-1556

[3] Syed SA, et al. A new experimental model: The vascular pedicle cutaneous flap over the dorsal aspect (flank and hip) of the rat. British Journal of Plastic Surgery. 1992;**45**(1):23-25

[4] Finseth F, Cutting C. An experimental neurovascular island skin flap for the study of the delay phenomenon. Plastic and Reconstructive Surgery. 1978;**61**(3):412-420

[5] Petry JJ, Wortham KA. The anatomy of the epigastric flap in the experimental rat. Plastic and Reconstructive Surgery. 1984;**74**(3):410-413

[6] Nishikawa H, Manek S, Green CJ. The oblique rat groin flap. British Journal of Plastic Surgery. 1991;**44**(4):295-298

[7] Koudsi B, Khouri RK. Thigh adductor flap: An experimental model for free flap transfer in the rat. Microsurgery. 1992;**13**(6):338-339

[8] Yim KK, et al. Microvascular transfer of anterior and posterior gracilis muscles in rats. Microsurgery. 1991;**12**(4):262-267

[9] Battal MN, et al. A new experimental model of a true myocutaneous flap in the rat: The gluteus maximus myocutaneous flap. The Journal of Reconstructive Microsurgery. 1997;**13**(4):251-255

[10] Black KS, et al. Two new composite tissue allograft models in rats to study neuromuscular functional return. Transplantation Proceedings. 1987;**19**(1 Pt 2):1118-1119

[11] Tonken HP, et al. Microvascular transplant of the gastrocnemius muscle in rats. Microsurgery. 1993;**14**(2):120-124

[12] Dogan T, et al. Quadriceps femoris muscle flap: Largest muscle flap model in the rat. The Journal of Reconstructive Microsurgery. 1999;**15**(6):433-437

[13] Bayramicli M. Experimental microsurgery (in Turkish). Istanbul, Argos iletisim; 2005

[14] Zhang F, et al. Pectoralis major muscle free flap in rat model. Microsurgery. 1994; **15**(12):853-856

[15] Tilgner A, Herrberger U, Oswald P. Myocutaneous flap models in the rat. Anatomy, histology and operative technique of the latissimus dorsi myocutaneous flap. Zeitschrift fur Versuchstierkunde. 1988;**31**(5):225-232

[16] Wan C, et al. Reducing the vascular delay period in latissimus dorsi muscle flaps for use in cardiomyoplasty. Plastic and Reconstructive Surgery. 2002;**109**(5):1630-1637

[17] Zhang F, et al. Microvascular transfer of the rectus abdominis muscle and myocutaneous flap in rats. Microsurgery. 1993;**14**(6):420-423

[18] Chen SG, et al. Free vascularized fibular bone flap in the rat. Microsurgery. 2000;**20**(1):1-5

Section 2

Perforator Flaps

Chapter 3

Perforator Flaps: Principles and Techniques

Goktekin Tenekeci

Additional information is available at the end of the chapter

http://dx.doi.org/10.5772/intechopen.71270

Abstract

Evolution of flaps has continued after the introduction of fasciocutaneous and musculocutaneous flaps. Perforator flaps have evolved, and they have provided many new flaps with new pedicles all over the body presenting important advantages. Better understanding of vascular anatomy and pattern of skin circulation has become possible by numerous cadaveric studies. As a result, widespread use of perforator flaps, either pedicled or free, has become possible. Perforator flaps have provided freedom of flap design with over 350 perforators all over the body, reliability, and reduced donor site morbidity. However, success begins with planning and continues with operative procedure. Here, in this relatively new field of reconstructive surgery, the following are discussed: the correct planning of perforator flaps, microanatomy of perforators, and what to do during the operation based on previous reports. Lastly, some brief information and examples of perforator-based workhorse flaps are given.

Keywords: perforator, flap

1. Introduction

Two main algorithms are applied for reconstruction of tissue defects: the reconstructive ladder and the reconstructive elevator systems. The philosophy of the reconstructive ladder system is to use the simplest possible reconstructive option to reconstruct the defect. According to the "reconstructive ladder" concept primary closure, skin graft, local flap, and lastly distant flap options are evaluated and used for reconstructing a defect. The simplest option to reconstruct a defect in this order is used. However, according to the reconstructive elevator system, patients' needs determine the reconstructive option to be used. In order to achieve a better functional and esthetic outcome, to improve donor site appearance, and to reduce its morbidity, many surgeons have used free flap transfer as the first choice over the past two decades [1]. Therefore, the reconstructive elevator system is favored since it is more functional and reduces donor site morbidity especially after the introduction of perforator-free flaps.

Modern technology has enabled us to produce finer microsurgical and surgical instruments; improvement in optics has produced improved operative microscopes [2]. Along with this, an increasing number of centers all over the world give microsurgical training opportunities, enabling more and more reconstructive surgeons to perform reconstructive microsurgical operations [2]. As a result of this, there is a general shift in favor of the reconstructive elevator versus the reconstructive ladder system all over the world. This means, more complicated operations that consider patients' future functionality and donor site morbidity are performed. Donor site morbidity does not always refer to donor site appearance but, more importantly, it refers to sacrification of important vessels, underlying muscle, etc. After the introduction of perforator flaps to the field of reconstructive surgery, harvest and use of perforator flaps as a new option has become popular because of its numerous advantages compared to more traditional flaps. These advantages include the reliability of perforator flaps, decrease in donor site morbidity when compared to nonperforator options, and the possibility to use each perforator flap as a local pedicled flap or as a free flap. As a result of this, perforator flaps have gained legitimate popularity all over the world. Radial forearm free flaps or latissimus dorsi free flaps can be given as examples for less frequently used reconstructive options after popularization of perforator based free flaps.

In the past, before perforator flaps gained popularity, random pattern flaps with no described or known vascular supply had been frequently used to reconstruct defects. Ponten has described various lengths to width ratios for random pattern flaps in different locations of the body. However, as a result of a better understanding of blood supply to skin, a new era has begun in the field of reconstructive surgery. This has led to the development and use of fasciocutaneous and musculocutaneous flaps supported by the "angiosome theory."

Evolution of flaps has continued contrary to the belief that there is very little left to discover about flap design [2]. In 1989, Koshima and Soeda reported on a skin flap supplied by a perforating vessel originating from the deep inferior epigastric artery and perforating the deep fascia [3]. This was the first perforator flap reported and was the beginning of another era in the field of reconstructive microsurgery. Following this report, an increasing number of papers have been reported sharing experience in reconstructing defects all over the body either by using local perforator flaps or by using perforator-free flaps.

2. Description, classification, and nomenclature of perforator flaps

In 2003, Blondeel et al. reported a paper representing the consensus of opinions of a group of pioneers in the field of perforator flap surgery that were reached during the Fifth International Course on Perforator Flaps in Gent in September 2001 [4]. They tried to classify perforators according to perforators' anatomy, the route they passed through until they reached the subcutaneous tissue by piercing the deep fascia. According to this paper, five types of perforators were defined: "(1) direct perforators: these perforated the deep fascia and supplied the subcutaneous tissue and skin, (2) indirect muscle perforators that gave muscular branches but predominantly supplied skin and subcutaneous tissue, (3) indirect muscle perforators that gave branches to muscle, predominantly supplied muscle but gave secondary branches to subcutaneous tissue, (4) indirect perimysial perforators that traveled within the perimysium between the muscle fibers before piercing the deep fascia, (5) indirect septal perforators that traveled between the intermuscular septum, and pierced the deep fascia and supplied the subcutaneous tissue and skin" [4]. After the "2001 consensus" in classification of perforators, Blondeel et al. reported on roundtable talks on flap terminology at the "Sixth International Course on Perforator Flaps" that was held in Taipei from October 23 until October 26, 2002. During this meeting, they tried to simplify perforator classification and reported this simplified consensus in 2003 [5]. According to this, flaps are classified under three types: "(1) indirect muscle perforators or myocutaneous perforators that traverse through muscle and perforate the outer layer of deep fascia to supply overlying skin, (2) indirect septal perforators or septocutaneous perforators that traverse septum and supply overlying skin after perforating the outer layer of deep fascia, and (3) direct perforators that perforate deep fascia only" [5]. If we look from a practical point of view, it is important to know what kind of dissection is to be made: an intramuscular dissection or a dissection for a septocutaneous perforator. Dissection of a septocutaneous perforator requires a tedious dissection but is easier when compared with the dissection of a musculocutaneous perforator. However, dissection of a musculocutaneous perforator requires experience and much care. From this point, it is important to distinguish between two. On the other hand, we believe it is also very important to know the subtypes of musculocutaneous perforators for academic purposes.

Another issue concerns the nomenclature of perforator flaps. In Gent, they tried to reach a consensus on the nomenclature of new perforator flaps. Until this time, same perforator flaps are being reported in articles or in scientific meetings under different names, and this causes confusion among readers or audients. For this reason, the following statement is accepted:

"A perforator flap should be named after the nutrient artery or vessels and not after the underlying muscle. If there is a potential to harvest multiple perforator flaps from one vessel, the name of each flap should be based on its anatomical region or muscle" [4].

3. Perforasome theory and perforator anatomy

Perforasome theory has been raised by Saint-Cyr et al. as a result of a cadaveric study [6]. This theory defines the perforators supplying skin, the microanatomy of perforating vessels, perfusion characteristics, and the relationship among neighboring perforators all around the body. This theory also gives us clues in correct designing of perforator flaps. The importance of direct and indirect linking vessels has also been shown in this study. Similarly, Taylor and Palmer have defined the angiosome concept; they have demonstrated that the whole body is divided into composite blocks of tissue supplied by source vessels and each neighboring tissue block and source vessels communicate with each other by means of anastomotic vessels [7, 8]. Both are quite important studies that try to find answers to similar questions and are milestones in understanding the vascularization of skin.

The term "perforasome" has been used by Saint-Cyr et al. to describe the vascular arterial territory supplied by an individual perforator [6]. Over 350 perforators exist throughout the body [6]. In order to correctly plan perforator flaps, we have to know the territory of each perforator, the direction along which the perforator branches travel, and the anastomoses of each perforator with its neighboring perforators. For this purpose, Saint-Cyr et al. have published a study performed on fresh human cadavers; this study is a milestone in understanding the microanatomy of perforators and provides valuable information on how to plan a perforator flap [6]. "It has been reported that each perforasome is linked to the adjacent perforasomes by "direct and indirect linking vessels" [6]. "Indirect linking vessels are effective in capturing adjacent perforasome by means of recurrent blood flow through subdermal plexus" [6]". Indirect linking vessels and the choke vessels of "angiosome theory" reported by Taylor et al. are the same [9]. According to Taylor et al., every angiosome is usually connected to other angiosomes by reduced caliber vessels named "choke vessels." "Direct linking vessels are larger vessels that link adjacent perforators resulting in capturing of neighboring perforasomes based on single perforator [6]." The synonym of direct linking vessels in perforasome theory is "true anastomosis." The vessel calibers of true anastomosis do not change and are especially found in places where vessels are accompanied by cutaneous nerves, in muscles, nerve trunks, or after flaps that have been delayed [10–15]. Therefore, knowledge about the direction along which direct and indirect linking vessels lie is very important to correctly plan perforator flaps because inclusion of direct and indirect perforators secures perforator flaps. Making sure to include direct and indirect linking vessels into the flap enables reconstructive microsurgeons to harvest a larger flap by incorporating neighboring perforasomes into the flap. "Flaps raised from the extremities should be designed parallel to the extremities since the direction of the linking vessels follow the axiality of the involved limb [6]." "However, flap design should be made perpendicular to the midline for flaps that will be harvested from the trunk since the axiality of the trunk follows the axiality of the muscle fibers of posterior trunk and chest, and this is perpendicular to the midline [6]." That is why long axis of anterolateral thigh flaps, posterior tibial artery perforator flaps, medial sural artery perforator flaps, and many other flaps raised on the extremities are planned parallel to the long axis of the extremity, whereas long axis of dorsal intercostal artery perforator flaps, lateral intercostal artery perforator flaps, thoracodorsal artery perforator flaps, and other perforator flaps harvested from trunk and chest wall are planned perpendicular to the midline and have a horizontal oblique direction.

"Vascular filling and density is highest in the perforasomes of perforators from the same source artery, but lower in the neighboring perforasomes of other perforators branching from different source arteries [6]." This is known as the "preferential filling" of perforasomes; preferential filling occurs in the perforators branching from the same source artery initially, but later occurs in the perforators branching from neighboring source arteries. Therefore, it may be concluded that a perforator flap carrying neighboring perforasomes arising from different source arteries harvested on a single perforator will have less perfusion than a flap harvested on single perforator carrying two adjacent perforasomes arising from the same source artery. For example, when a large thoracodorsal artery perforator flap is planned, it must be planned over the latissimus dorsi muscle to incorporate neighboring perforasomes of other perforators arising from the thoracodorsal artery. It must be remembered that if perforasomes of dorsal intercostal artery perforators or circumflex scapular artery perforators

http://dx.doi.org/10.5772/intechopen.71270

are to be incorporated instead of perforasomes of thoracodorsal artery perforators, the vascular filling pressure of that flap may be less in the perforasomes of other source arteries. This is very important in flap planning.

"Perforators found close to an articulation have a flow distribution away from this articulation [6]." "However, perforators found at a midpoint between two articulations or found at the midpoint of trunk have multidirectional flow distribution [6]." Planning of posterior tibial artery perforator flaps are good examples of perforators found close to articulations. Distal perforators of posterior tibial artery arise 9–12 cm proximal to the medial malleolus of tibia at the ankle joint [16]. Skin island of posterior tibial artery perforator flaps supplied by distal perforators of posterior tibial artery must be planned toward the proximal part of cruris (away from the articulation). On the other hand, perforators of anterolateral thigh flaps arise around the midpoint of the line drawn between anterior superior iliac spine and the superolateral part of patella. That is why, anterolateral thigh flaps may be planned proximal to and distal to the perforator due to the multidirectional flow.

4. Harvesting a perforator flap

Advantages of perforator flaps include the potential to harvest flaps based on any reliable perforator throughout the body that they do not sacrifice major vessels since they are supplied by the branches of these vessels and that they do not necessarily sacrifice muscle if muscle is not needed for reconstruction. In radial forearm flaps, the radial artery is incorporated. Therefore, after the radial forearm flap has been harvested, the whole hand is supplied by ulnar artery only. Sacrification of an artery such as the radial artery is believed to produce considerable morbidity. On the other hand, when perforator flaps are used, the source artery can be preserved. In case of a musculocutaneous perforator, intramuscular dissection may become challenging. However, if intramuscular pedicle dissection is performed, sacrification of muscle can be avoided. For instance, when a thoracodorsal artery perforator flap is being harvested based on a musculocutaneous perforator, intramuscular dissection must be performed in order to preserve underlying muscle namely latissimus dorsi muscle in this example. The same is true for anterolateral thigh flaps whenever the flap is supplied by a musculocutaneous perforator. However, if needed, such as in the obliteration of a dead space, a muscle cuff can be incorporated into the harvested flap based on a separate perforator.

Tedious dissection is very important in perforator flap harvest. It must be performed under loupe magnification and requires special expertise and experience. Especially, intramuscular perforator dissection can be challenging. That is why, perforator flap harvesting requires a learning curve. For beginners of perforator flap dissection, a detailed anatomy of the perforator flap being harvested must be known and training in one of the experienced centers on perforator flap dissection is strongly recommended.

There is a conflict about the skeletonization of the perforators supplying perforator flaps. Some groups claim that skeletonization of perforators supplying local perforator flaps is not needed, whereas some others, including us, believe that without skeletonization of perforators, flap harvest is not completed. Groups who do not skeletonize perforating vessels claim that skeletonization of perforators is not performed in order to reduce the risk of damage to the perforating artery and its venae commitantes [17]. We believe that complete skeletonization of perforator is required, since soft tissue and fibrous bands around perforators may cause compression of perforating artery and venae commitantes, thus causing venous insufficiency and/or arterial compromise of perforator flaps. Therefore, we believe that it is a "must" in perforator dissection. We know that skin is supplied by rich vascular plexuses including subepidermal plexus, dermal plexus, subdermal plexus, subcutaneous plexus, prefascial plexus, and subfascial plexus. All these plexuses contribute to the vascularization of skin. Our opinion is to harvest the flap with the fascia overlying the muscle because it is important in vascularization of the harvested flap. This is especially so, when a large flap is being harvested since prefascial and subfascial plexuses will be left intact on the harvested flap.

5. Flap circulation

Flap circulation is a dynamic process. Therefore, cadaveric studies are not sufficient to help us understand the exact margins a perforator can supply. It must be remembered that when all the side branches (muscle and cutaneous branches) of a perforator emanating from the source artery are ligated, hyperperfusion of the flap pedicle will occur [6]. Hyperperfusion of the perforator artery and its increased vascular filling cause its dilatation [6]. This, in turn, will open up the anastomotic vessels, namely direct and indirect linking vessels, and result in perfusion of adjacent perforasomes belonging to neighboring perforators [6]. Choke vessels (synonymous with indirect linking vessels) dilate as much as true anastomosis size; however, this takes 2–3 days [12, 13]. During this time, hyperplasia, elongation, and hypertrophy of cells in the tunica intima, media, and adventitia occur. This leads to the thinning of vessel walls, followed by thickening by the seventh day [13]. However, if necrosis occurs, it usually takes place in this anastomotic zone. Perfusion pressure decreases, arteriovenous shunting occurs, and oxygen tension is subsequently lowered during the first 3–4 days, a process that leads to necrosis [18, 19].

There are over 350 perforators throughout the body [6]. Perforator flaps can be potentially harvested from anywhere, where there is a reliable perforator. Perforator flaps can be used as local perforator flaps or as perforator-free flaps. With the report of freestyle free flaps by Wei and Mardini [20], a new gate has been opened for reconstruction of defects using tissues harvested from anywhere of the body provided that tissue encountered is "the most suitable and similar" and is supplied by a reliable perforator. However, freestyle perforator flaps can also be used as local options for soft tissue reconstruction. For local perforator flaps, defect-perforator distance, reliability of perforator, scar tissue around the perforator, and over the planned flap (if there is) must all be considered. As mentioned before, perforator flaps can be used as local perforator flaps or as perforator-free flaps. Perforator-free flaps require vascular anastomosis onto the source vessels or onto other perforating vessels in the recipient site, whereas local perforator flaps do not. Therefore, the dissection part of the operation is similar

http://dx.doi.org/10.5772/intechopen.71270

in local perforator flaps and perforator-free flaps. However, in order to cover the defect, local perforator flaps are mobilized in a propeller, rotational, advancement, or transpositional movement fashion. Perforator free flaps require vascular anastomosis; therefore, a longer operation is performed. Correct planning of perforator flaps is of primary importance for the success of flaps. Perforators supplying perforator flaps have a static zone and a dynamic zone. The static zone is the zone supplied by the perforator itself, whereas the dynamic zone is the zone a perforator can supply beyond its own perforasome. This means that the dynamic zone is the potential zone of a perforator to supply the perforasomes of neighboring perforators. Saint-Cyr et al. reported that vascular filling of perforators from the same source artery is more, when compared to vascular filling of neighboring perforators from different source arteries, and this is explained by "preferential filling" [6]. Therefore, a perforator flap planned incorporating perforasomes of perforators arising from the same source artery may be safer than that combining perforasomes of perforators from different source arteries. For the same reason, after identifying a large perforator at the desired flap base, Taylor et al. [21] look for another perforator close to the first perforator in all radial directions and combine both perforators on a line drawn in between; this line is going to be the flap axis. They believe that this kind of flap planning is safe [21]. The anatomical territory of a cutaneous perforator is defined as the zone that connects the perforator with adjacent perforators in all directions and is separated from the anatomical zones of other perforators by the anastomotic zone between each anatomical territory. On the other hand, the clinical territory of each perforator is wider than its particular anatomical territory as it usually captures the neighboring anatomical territory of the neighboring perforator. It may even capture the anatomical territory of the one beyond, especially when perforators are linked together by true anastomosis or direct linking vessels [7].

6. Assessment of perforator location

Taylor et al. have reported that locating perforators correctly in well-muscled volunteers using a handheld Doppler is comparable with the location of corresponding perforators found in fresh cadavers after dissection and concluded that there was a close correlation [22]. However, investigation in this issue continued. Color Doppler ultrasound and computed tomography angiography (CT angiography) is frequently performed for this purpose. Feng et al. have compared color Doppler ultrasound and CT angiography for their reliability and sensitivity in detecting the location of perforators accurately [23]. They have reported that, preoperative color Doppler ultrasound (95%) is more accurate with respect to CT angiography (82.5%) in detecting the localization of dominant perforators. However, this difference has not been statistically significant. The results obtained with Color Doppler Ultrasound has a mean error of 1.11 ± 1.29 mm, whereas CT angiography has a mean error of 2.55 ± 2.63 mm, a statistically significant difference. On the other hand, the time needed to evaluate the images using CT angiography (27.2 ± 1.77 minutes) has been less than those used for color Doppler ultrasound (34.83 ± 3.55 minutes). The success of color Doppler ultrasound has been directly related to the experience of radiologist; however, the same has not been true for CT angiography [23]. Metal implants are known to cause artifact formation in CT angiography images; however, this does not apply to color Doppler ultrasound. On the other hand, compared to CT angiography, Doppler ultrasound is a cheaper modality [23]. As a result, Feng et al. have advocated the use of color Doppler ultrasound in experienced hands instead of CT angiography for more correctly locating perforators, and also, it is less expensive [23].

7. Risk factors of perforator flaps

In order to identify risk factors of perforator propeller flaps in lower extremity defects, Bekara et al. searched MEDLINE, PubMedCentral, Embase, and Cochrane databases for reported series of lower extremity reconstruction using pedicled perforator propeller flaps between 1991 and 2004 [24]. In total, 428 perforator propeller flaps from 40 articles which performed for lower extremity reconstruction were included in the study [24]. Partial necrosis was found in 10.2%, whereas total flap necrosis was found in 3.5% of cases [24]. Patients older than 60, or patients who had diabetes or arteriopathy, were determined as significant risk factors for flap failure [24]. However, smoking, acute injury, post-traumatic injury, location of defect over the distal third of lower leg, inclusion of fascia, pedicle rotation greater than 120°, accompanying bone fracture, and surface area greater than 100 cm^2 were found to have no significant effect on flap success [24]. Hypertension could not be evaluated due to lack of data [24]. Since this study was a meta-analysis, it had some limitations, however: lack of standardization (different surgical techniques and different approaches by different surgeons, and flaps used for reconstruction), missing data (comorbidity, localization, size of flap, cause, pedicle rotation), and including nonhomogenous patient groups [24]. Nevertheless, it is important to identify risk factors threatening perforator flap viability since patients are to be selected considering those risk factors along with many other factors. Another important issue that must be considered in reconstructive planning is defect etiology. In traumatic defects, post-traumatic vessel disease may have developed [25]. "Post-traumatic vessel disease is defined as progressive changes in vessel and perivascular tissues following trauma" [24] and "loss of normal easy dissection planes, around the vessels, loss of vasa vasorum, increased tendency of vessels to vasospasm or easily damaging vessels during dissection along with lack of thromboresistant properties of healthy vessels" [24]. Therefore, post-traumatic vessel disease is considered as a risk factor in reconstructive surgery, and the reconstructive surgeon must be aware of this. Because of this, the reconstructive surgeon must be familiar with problem solving and must have a special strategy for each case, individualizing each patient during reconstructive planning.

Brief information about some of the workhorse flaps and some case examples will be given in the following section.

8. The anterolateral thigh flap

The anterolateral thigh flap is probably the most commonly used perforator flap for reconstruction of soft tissue defects especially when transferred as a free flap. The anterolateral thigh

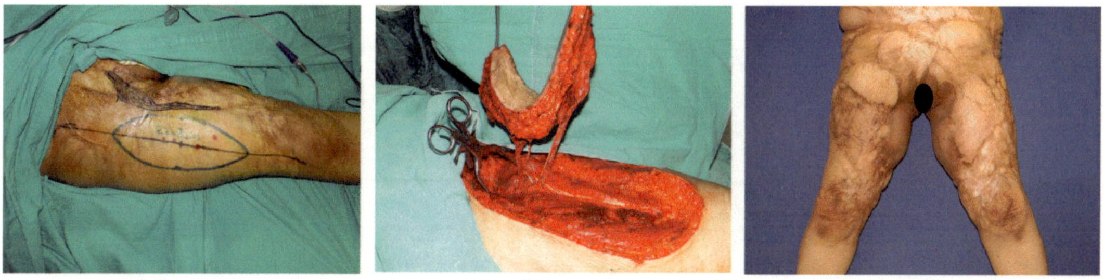

(a) (b) (c)

Figure 1. (a) The patient is feeling discomfort standing upright because of unstable scarring and a slight contracture over the right inguinal region. The operative plan is to excise the contracture band and reconstruct the defect using a pedicled anterolateral thigh flap. (b) The anterolateral thigh flap has been elevated. Note that two pedicles supplying the flap have been dissected off. (c) Patient as seen 18 months postoperatively. Note that patient can easily abduct and extend her thighs.

flap is supplied by the descending branch of lateral circumflex femoral artery, which is the branch of deep femoral artery [26]. A straight line is drawn from the anterior superior iliac spine to the superolateral edge point of patella [26]. The flap pedicle lies between rectus femoris and vastus lateralis [26]. The perforator supplying this flap can be septocutaneous or musculocutaneous. The anterolateral thigh flap has a long pedicle that is a great advantage for use as a free flap or for use in reconstruction of locoregional defects (**Figure 1**). It can be harvested with a muscle cuff or with fascia according to patients' needs [27]. This flap can be raised with a muscle cuff from vastus lateralis muscle as a chimeric flap [28] or with fascia lata for different reconstructive purposes [29].

9. The thoracodorsal artery perforator flap

The source vessel for the thoracodorsal artery perforator flap is the thoracodorsal artery. This artery is a branch of the subscapular system and divides into transverse and descending branches after entering to the latissimus dorsi muscle. According to the cadaveric dissections of Heitmann et al. investigating the anatomical basis of thoracodorsal artery perforator flaps, out of 20 specimens, a total of 64 musculocutaneous perforators larger than 0.5 mm were found [30]. In total, 36 of these perforators were arising from the descending branch whereas 28 were arising from the transverse branch [30]. However, in 11 dissections, there was also a direct cutaneous branch with an extravascular course [30]. The flap is raised in the lateral decubitus position, and an incision lateral to the lateral border of latissimus dorsi muscle is made [31] (**Figure 2**). After the perforator is found, dissection of the perforator is continued until adequate length is reached. However, during dissection of the flap, attention must be paid for preservation of the thoracodorsal nerve [31]. In addition to their local use, thoracodorsal artery perforator flaps are also favorable flaps for transfer as free flaps taking advantage of their long pedicle.

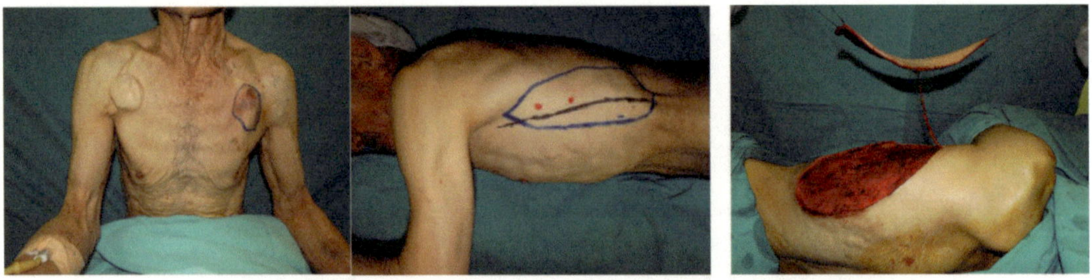

(a) (b)

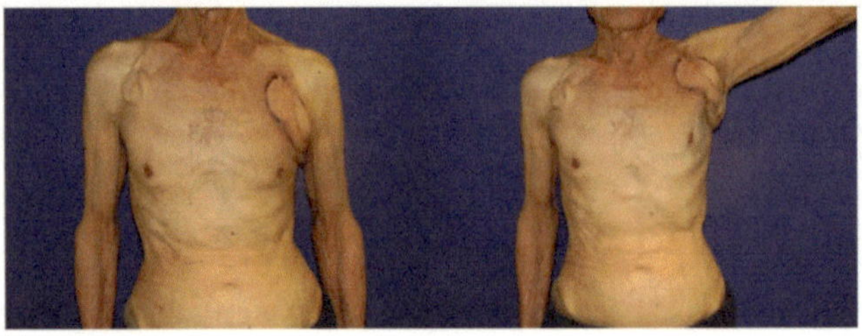

(c)

Figure 2. (a) An exposed pacemaker is seen over the left pectoral region. The operative plan is to excise the infected skin and reconstruct the defect using a thoracodorsal artery perforator flap. Flap planning is seen. A 9 × 9 cm defect is formed after excision and flap dimensions are 20 × 9 cm. (b) The thoracodorsal artery perforator flap has been elevated. (c) Patient as seen 3 months postoperatively.

10. Superior gluteal artery perforator flap

Koshima et al. were probably the first to report on the use of gluteal artery perforator flaps for reconstruction of sacral pressure sores [32]. Superior gluteal artery perforator flaps can be used in soft tissue reconstruction of locoregional defects as well as in breast reconstruction when used as free flaps [33]. However, for use in breast reconstruction, they are usually indicated in those whom abdominal flaps are risky or cannot be used [31]. Usually, three perforators supply superior gluteal artery perforator flaps [31]. Superior gluteal artery perforators are found one-third of the distance along the line drawn from the posterior superior iliac spine to the greater trochanter [31]. After the localization of the pedicle using a handheld Doppler, the flap may be centered on that pedicle or may be designed eccentrically. After the incisions have been made and the perforator supplying the flap has been found, intramuscular dissection toward the sacrum is performed in order to elongate the flap pedicle (**Figure 3**). Dissection of a single perforator is adequate to supply the flap. However, one can dissect more than one perforator to supply the flap. The donor area can be closed primarily.

11. Conclusion

Perforator flaps have evolved as a result of better understanding of the dynamics of the vascular supply and drainage as well as the vascular microanatomy of flaps. Perforator flaps are a step forward in reconstruction of soft tissue defects; they have opened a new era in

http://dx.doi.org/10.5772/intechopen.71270

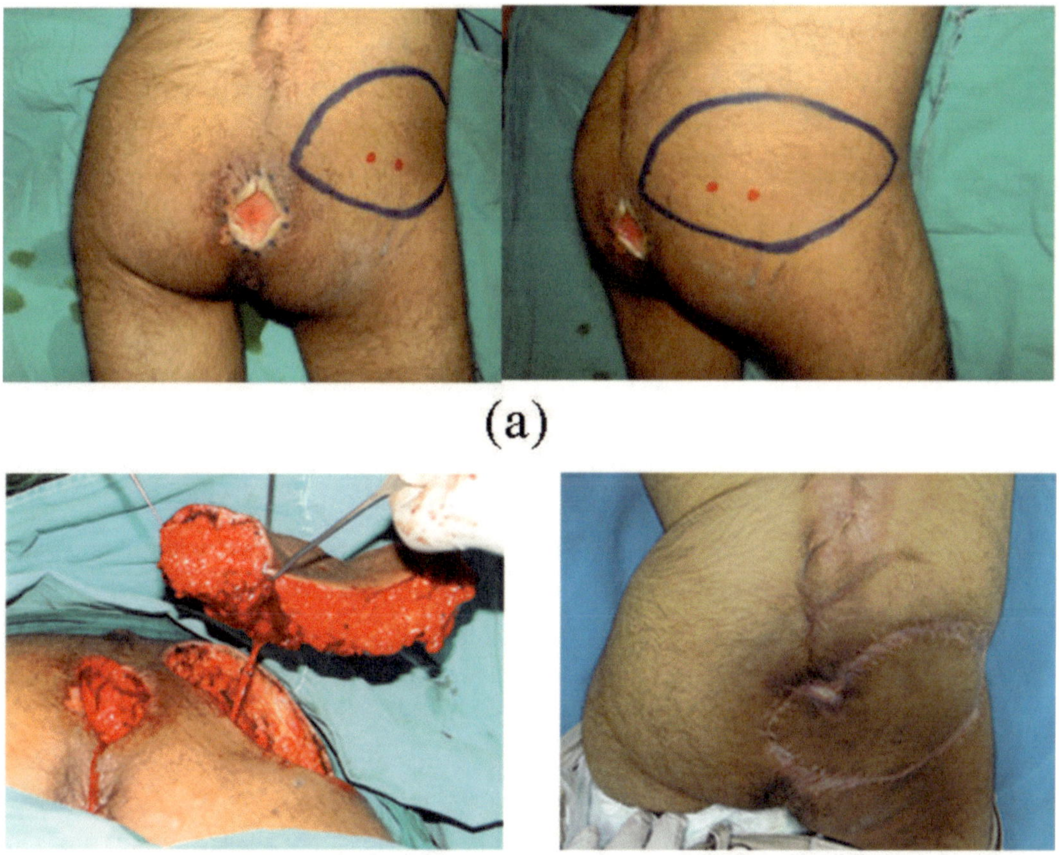

(a) (b) (c)

Figure 3. (a) A presacral pressure sore is seen in a previously operated meningomyelocele patient. The operative plan is to reconstruct the defect using a superior gluteal artery perforator flap. The defect size is 4.5 × 5.5 cm and the planned flap is 16 × 8.5 cm. (b) The superior gluteal artery perforator flap has been elevated based on a single perforator. (c) The patient following reconstruction as seen 1 year postoperatively. Note that a small area of recurrence is seen at the superior border of the flap after 1 year.

reconstructive surgery. Perforator flaps provide very important advantages in reconstructive surgery. Nevertheless, they are not without hazards. For this reason, risk factors in perforator flap surgery and clues to successful planning must be kept in mind while planning reconstruction using perforator flaps.

Author details

Goktekin Tenekeci

Address all correspondence to: dr_tenekecig@hotmail.com

Department of Plastic, Reconstructive and Aesthetic Surgery, Mersin University Hospital, Mersin, Turkey

References

[1] Engel H, Lin CH, Wei FC. Role of microsurgery in lower extremity reconstruction. Plastic and Reconstructive Surgery. 2011;**127**(1S):228S-238S

[2] Blondeel P, Hallock G, Morris SF, Neligan PC. Perforator Flaps: Anatomy, Technique & Clinical Applications. St. Louis: Quality Medical Publishing Inc; 2006

[3] Koshima I, Soeda S. Inferior epigastric artery skin flap without rectus abdominis muscle. British Journal of Plastic Surgery. 1989;**42**:645

[4] Blondeel PN, Van Landuyt KH, Monstrey SJ, et al. The "gent" consensus on perforator flap terminology: Preliminary definitions. Plastic and Reconstructive Surgery. 2003;**112**(5): 1378-1383

[5] Blondeel PN, Van Landuyt K, Hamdi M, Monstrey SJ. Perforator flap terminology: Update 2002. Clinics in Plastic Surgery. 2003;**30**:343-346

[6] Saint-Cyr M, Wong C, Schaverien M, et al. The perforasome theory: Vascular anatomy and clinical implications. Plastic and Reconstructive Surgery. 2009;**124**(5):1529-1544

[7] Taylor GI, Corlett RJ, Dhar SC, Ashton MW. The anatomical (angiosome) and clinical territories of cutaneous perforating arteries: Development of the concept and designing safe flaps. Plastic and Reconstructive Surgery. 2011;**127**(4):1447-1459

[8] Taylor GI, Palmer JH. The vascular territories (angiosomes) of the body: Experimental study and clinical applications. British Journal of Plastic Surgery. 1987;**40**:113-141

[9] Lecours C, Saint-Cyr M, Wong C, et al. Freestyle pedicle perforator flaps: Clinical results and vascular anatomy. Plastic and Reconstructive Surgery. 2010;**126**(5):1589-1603

[10] Taylor GI, Corlett RJ. The cutaneous vascular territories in pig and man. Paper Presented at: ASPRS Meeting. New York, NY: Surgical Forum No. 67; 1981

[11] Callegari PR, Taylor GI, Caddy C, et al. An anatomic review of the delay phenomenon: I. Experimental studies. Plastic and Reconstructive Surgery. 1992;**89**:397-407

[12] Morris SF, Taylor GI. Predicting the survival of experimental skin flaps based on a knowledge of the vascular architecture. Plastic and Reconstructive Surgery. 1993;**92**:1352-1371

[13] Dhar S, Taylor GI. The delay phenomenon: The story unfolds. Plastic and Reconstructive Surgery. 1999;**104**:2079-2091

[14] Taylor GI, Corlett RJ, Caddy CM, Zelt RG. An anatomic review of the delay phenomenon: II. Clinical applications. Plastic and Reconstructive Surgery. 1992;**89**:408-416

[15] Taylor GI. The delayed TRAM flap for breast reconstruction: Why, when and how. Operative Techniques in Plastic and Reconstructive Surgery. 1999;**6**:74-82

[16] Chan Wei F. Flaps and Reconstructive Surgery. China: Elsevier; 2009

[17] Shin IS, Lee DW, Rah DK, Lee WJ. Reconstruction of pretibial defect using pedicled perforator flaps. Archives of Plastic Surgery. 2012;**39**(4):360-366

[18] Boyd BJ, Markland B, Dorion D, Pang CY, Morris S. Surgical augmentation of skin blood flow and viability in a pig musculocutaneous flap model. Plastic and Reconstructive Surgery. 1990;**86**:731-738

[19] Dorion D, Boyd JB, Pang CY. Augmentation of transmidline skin perfusion and viability in transverse rectus abdominis myocutaneous (TRAM) flaps in pigs. Plastic and Reconstructive Surgery. 1991;**88**:642-649

[20] Wei FC, Mardini S. Free-style free flaps. Plastic and Reconstructive Surgery. 2004;**114**:910-916

[21] Taylor GI, Gianoutsos MP, Morris SF. The neurovascular territories of the skin and muscles anatomic study and clinical implications. Plastic and Reconstructive Surgery. 1994;**94**:1-36

[22] Taylor GI, Doyle M, McCarten G. The Doppler probe for planning flaps: Anatomical study and clinical applications. British Journal of Plastic Surgery. 1990;**43**:1-16

[23] Feng S, Min P, Grasetti L, et al. A prospective head-to-head comparison of color doppler ultrasound and computed tomographic angiography in the preoperative planning of lower extremity perforator flaps. Plastic and Reconstructive Surgery. 2016;**137**(1):335-347

[24] Bekara F, Herlin C, Mojollal A, et al. A systematic review and meta-analysis of perforator-pedicled propeller flaps in lower extremity defects: Identification of risk factors for complications. Plastic and Reconstructive Surgery. 2016;**137**(1):314-331

[25] Acland RD. Refinements in lower extremity free flap surgery. Clinics in Plastic Surgery. 1990;**17**:733-744

[26] DC X, Zhong SZ, Kong JM, et al. Applied anatomy of the anterolateral femoral flap. Plastic and Reconstructive Surgery. 1988;**82**:305-310

[27] Mohan AT, Sur YJ, Zhu L, et al. The concepts of propeller, perforator, keystone, and other local flaps and their role in the evolution of reconstruction. Plastic and Reconstructive Surgery. 2016;**138**(4):710-729

[28] Ozkan O, Ozkan O, Derin AT, et al. True functional reconstruction of total or subtotal glossectomy defects using a chimeric anterolateral thigh flap with both sensorial and motor innervation. Annals of Plastic Surgery. 2015;**74**(5):557-564

[29] Yildirim S, Taylan G, Akoz T. Use of fascia component of the anterolateral thigh flap for different reconstructive purposes. Annals of Plastic Surgery. 2005;**55**(5):479-484

[30] Heitmann C, Guerra A, Metzinger SW, et al. The thoracodorsal artery perforator flap: Anatomic basis and clinical application. Annals of Plastic Surgery. 2003;**51**(1):23-29

[31] Saint-Cyr M, Schaverien MV, Rohrich RJ. Perforator flaps: History, controversies, physiology, anatomy, and use in reconstruction. Plastic and Reconstructive Surgery. 2009;**123**(4):132-145

[32] Koshima I, Moriguchi T, Soeda S, et al. The gluteal perforator-based flap for repair of sacral pressure sores. Plastic and Reconstructive Surgery. 1993;**91**:678-683

[33] Guerra AB, Allen RJ, Dupin CL. Breast reconstruction with the superior gluteal artery perforator (S-GAP) flap. Seminars in Plastic Surgery. 2002;**16**:27-34

Chapter 4

Application of Free Flow-Through Anterolateral Thigh Flap for the Reconstruction of an Extremity Soft Tissue Defect Requiring Vascularization

Masaki Fujioka

Additional information is available at the end of the chapter

http://dx.doi.org/10.5772/intechopen.69404

Abstract

Patients with severe injury or vasculopathy of the extremities often require resurfacing of tissue defects as well as preservation of functional blood flow to distal areas. In conventional free flap transfer, the recipient vessel is sacrificed to facilitate pedicle anastomosis. On the other hand, a flow-through flap can provide blood flow to distal tissues. In this chapter, we present cases of successful salvage and reconstruction of the extremities using free flow-through flaps and highlight their advantages and applications. Free flow-through flap use should be a good option in the following cases: (1) Gustilo-Anderson IIIC type open fracture, (2) chronic ulcer resurfacing in the less vascularized extremities, and (3) additional blood supply for an ischemic flap. This flap facilitates not only the reconstruction of soft tissue defects, but also restores the functional vascular anatomy and maintains the original blood flow by interposing the T-portion of the vessel. This technique enables both vascular and soft tissue reconstructions simultaneously with minimal donor site problems. The anterolateral thigh flap is recommended as a free flow-through-type flap due to its advantages, including the variety of flap sizes, adequate calibers of the vascular pedicle, and the lack of a need for position changing.

Keywords: reconstruction of the extremity, soft tissue defects, revascularization, free flow-through flap, anterolateral thigh flap

1. Introduction

The disadvantage of traditional methods for reconstruction of soft tissue deficits using pedicle flaps is the need for multiple stages. In addition, donor site morbidity may be another disadvantage [1]. Following recent trends to overcome these problems, microsurgical flap transfer has revolutionized the reconstruction of soft tissue defects and has become a standard technique for the resurfacing of wounds, because it facilitates not only the safe coverage of large tissue defects, but also yields a cosmetically acceptable appearance [2–4]. Regarding hand and leg salvage and reconstruction after trauma and oncologic resection, surgeons often need to ensure both soft tissue coverage and blood flow supply to the distal extremities. Free tissue transfer can be superior to pedicle flap coverage for the resurfacing of a large tissue defect, as it reduces infection, induces bony healing, and optimizes limb salvage [5–7].

However, in conventional free flap transfer, the recipient vessel is sacrificed to facilitate pedicle anastomosis, a procedure which may reduce the distal blood flow. Especially, patients with vascular injury or chronic vasculopathy of the extremities require resurfacing of tissue defects as well as preservation of functional blood flow to distal areas. The concept of flow-through circulation in free flaps is using a one-staged technique for wound coverage and the revascularization of ischemic extremities [8].

In this chapter, several cases of successful salvage and extremity reconstruction using free flow-through flaps are presented; their advantages and applications are highlighted.

2. Surgical principle of free flow-through flap

In the flow-through flap concept, both the proximal and distal ends of the vascular pedicle of a free flap are anastamosed to provide blood flow to distal tissues (**Figure 1**). Since the concept

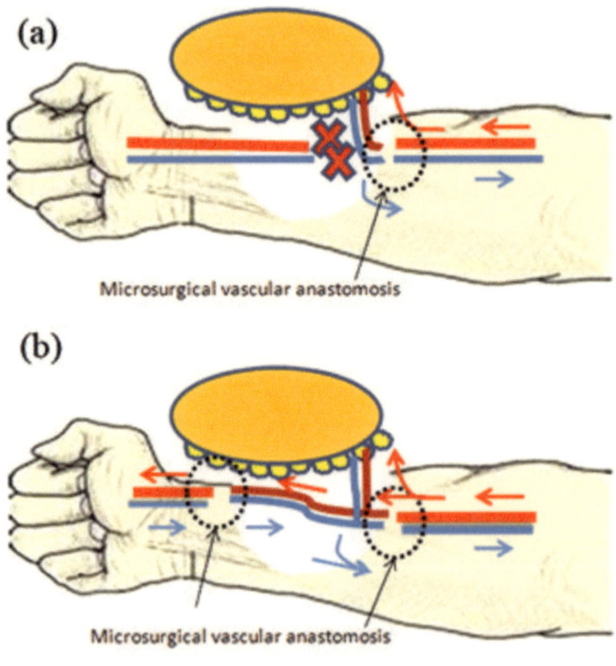

Figure 1. Schematic representation of the conventional and flow-through-type free flap. (a) Conventional free flap transfer. Major blood vessels are sacrificed; consequently, blood flow to the distal area is reduced. (b) Free flow-through flap transfer. Flow-through anastomosis preserves the recipient arterial flow, and the flaps are anatomically consistent.

was first described by Soutar et al. [9] using a radial forearm flap, many investigators have described the application of flow-through flaps for extremity reconstruction; latissimus dorsi musculocutaneous, rectus abdominis musculocutaneous, fibula osteomyocutaneous, and anterolateral thigh (ALT) flaps have been diversely used [9–12]. The ALT flap, in particular, can provide a large skin paddle yet with minimal donor site morbidity; thus, it is ideal for extremity reconstruction [10, 13–16].

3. Surgical procedure of free flow-through ALT flap

The musculofasciocutaneous ALT flap is supplied by the descending branch of the lateral femoral circumflex artery. Thus, it can be harvested as a fasciocutaneous or myocutaneous flap [17]. The descending branch traverses downward in the intermuscular septum between the rectus femoris and vastus lateralis muscle [18]. The rectus femoris muscle is retraced medially to expose the vascular bundle of the descending branch, and the length and diameter are examined. It proceeds downward, while sending perforators to supply the skin and muscles around the anterolateral aspect of the thigh (**Figure 2**). Usually, the descending branch has an external diameter of more than 2 mm at the proximal end with a pedicle of more than 8 cm in length (**Figure 3**) [18, 19]. When a larger flap is required, more than two perforator arteries should be preserved between the flap and pedicle.

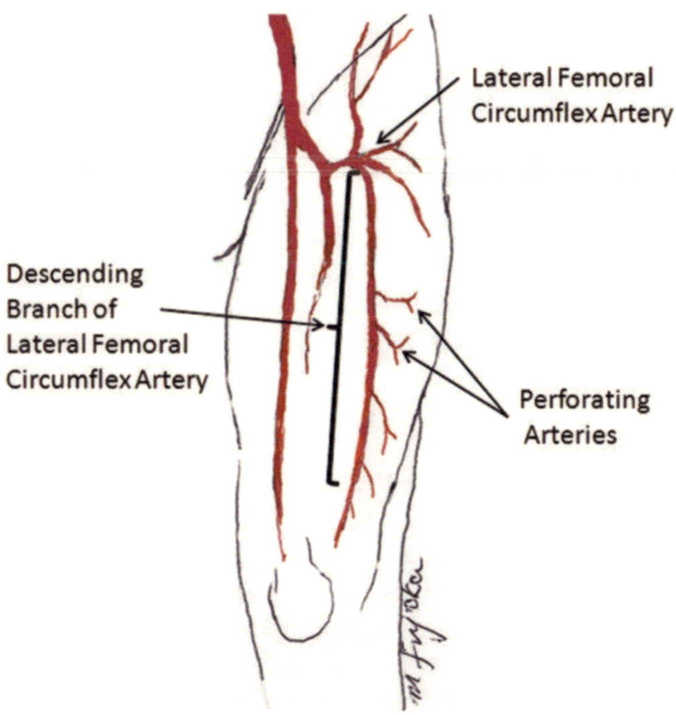

Figure 2. Vascular anatomy of the descending branch of the lateral femoral circumflex artery. The descending branch of the lateral femoral circumflex artery (marked in the illustration) is used as an interposing vessel.

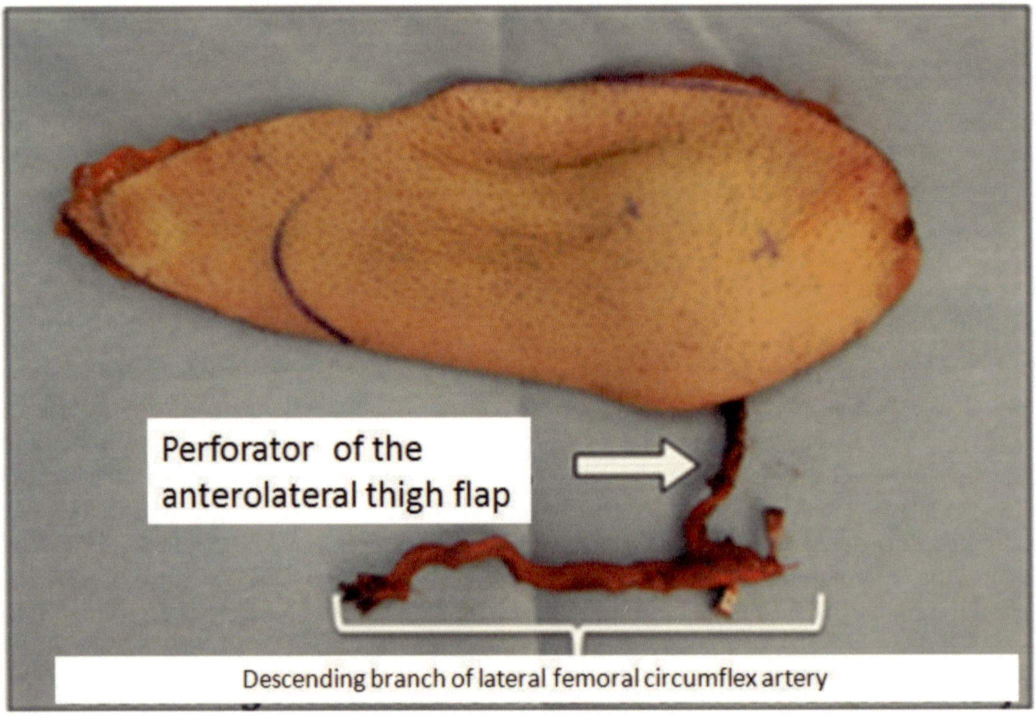

Figure 3. The harvested TFL flap and descending branch of the lateral femoral circumflex artery.

After the ALT flap has been harvested with an elliptical skin island from the thigh in the usual manner, the T-portion of the descending branch is interposed with the defect of the recipient artery (**Figure 1 (b)**). After confirming the vascular flow in the distal extremity, two veins are connected by end-to-end anastomosis. Vessel size mismatch has not been an issue because the caliber of the descending pedicle is considered to be consistently maintained throughout its course down the upper half to two-thirds of the vastus lateralis [20]. Generally, venous anastomosis does not have to be performed using the flow-through technique, except in re-plantation surgery for amputated limbs. Consequently, the interrupted recipient artery resumes normal blood flow, while the flap is vascularized via the perforator vessels of the descending branch.

4. Indication of free flow-through flap

Maintaining distal blood supply is important at all times for preventing the development of many diseases due to ischemia or peripheral circulation disorders (including frostbite, a contaminated leg ulcer, peripheral arterial disease, and skin and soft tissue problems associated with diabetes mellitus). Therefore, free flow-through flap use can be recommended in any case when combined free flap reconstruction and preservation/restoration of distal blood flow are required. In this fact indicating that the absolute indication of free flow-through flap use may be limited. However, additional indications include severe trauma involving the extremities and after malignant tumor resection, as these often cause blood vessel loss associated with soft tissue defects. Extremity reconstruction in vasculopathy patients also requires primary preservation of functional blood flow to distal areas. In such cases, one-stage reconstruction using a free flow-through flap may be an absolute application.

Free flow-through flap use should be a good option for soft tissue reconstruction in the following three cases:

(1) severe trauma (for example, Gustilo-Anderson IIIC type open fracture);

(2) chronic ulcer resurfacing in the less vascularized extremities; and

(3) additional blood supply for an ischemic flaps.

The author presents some cases of successful salvage and reconstruction of the extremities using free flow-through flaps.

5. Case presentation

5.1. Severe trauma (Gustilo-Anderson IIIC type open fracture)

Gustilo-Anderson IIIC type fracture requires both vascular and soft tissue repair immediately [21]. For reconstruction, flow-through flap use is beneficial, because blood flow of the distal extremity can be maintained, while the soft-tissue-insufficient wound can be resurfaced simultaneously.

Case 1. Due to a traffic accident, a 64-year-old man sustained a Gustilo-Anderson Type IIIC bone-exposing fracture to the left fibula and tibia with wide skin abrasion and involvement of the anterior tibial muscles (**Figure 4 (a, b)**). Circulation of the left foot had ceased because three main arteries in the leg (peroneal, posterior tibial, and anterior tibial arteries) had been ruptured with subsequent flow interruption (**Figure 5**). After the crushed bones had undergone external fixation, the bone-exposing wound was repaired with a free flow-through ALT flap. The T-portion of the descending branch of the ALT flap was interposed to the defect of the anterior tibial artery (**Figures 6, 7**). Subsequently, the interrupted anterior tibia artery resumed normal blood flow. The viability of the flap was favorable without infection or necrosis (**Figure 8**). The patient could walk without canes 1 year after surgery.

5.2. Chronic ulcer resurfacing in the less vascularized extremities

Chronic ulcer resurfacing, especially reconstruction after oncologic resection, in the less vascularized extremities is a challenge, because single artery scarification can cause amputation [22]. Free flow-through flap use is beneficial as it can maintain the distal blood flow [6].

Case 2. A 65-year-old man suffered from a chronic right leg ulcer, which rapidly enlarged and developed a fungating wound over a 6-month duration (**Figure 9**). Histological analysis of

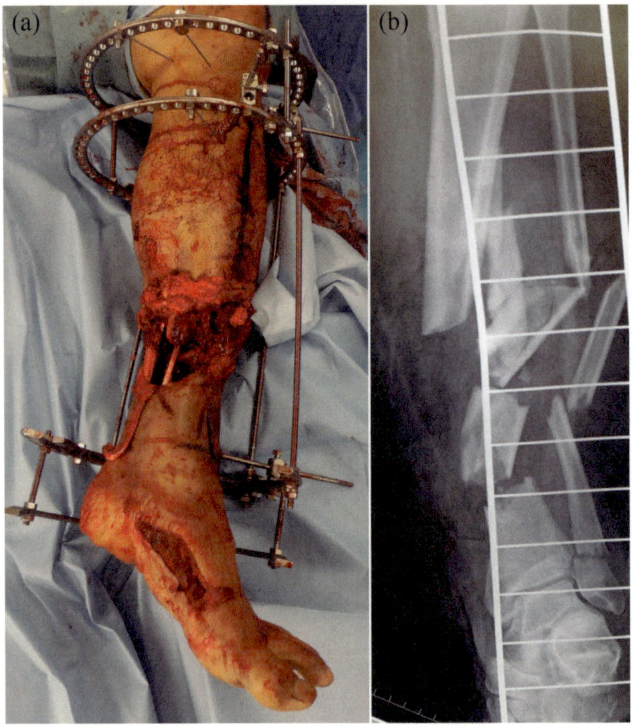

Figure 4. *Case 1.* The photographs show a Gustilo-Anderson IIIC type bone-exposing fracture to the left fibula and tibia with severe abrasion of the skin and anterior tibial muscles.

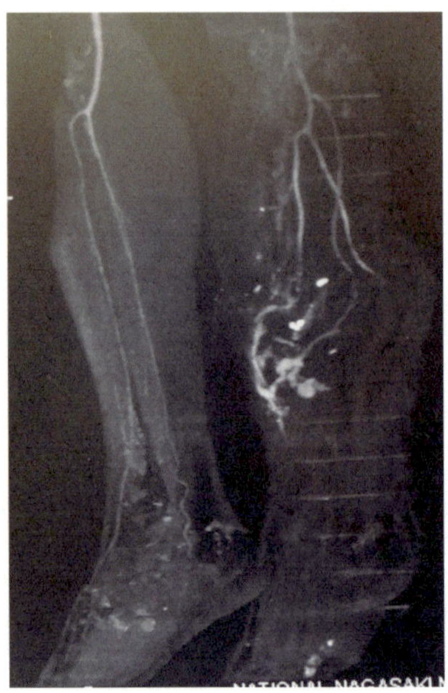

Figure 5. Contrast-enhanced CT reveals that circulation of the left foot had ceased because peroneal, posterior tibial, and involvement of anterior tibial arteries had been interrupted.

http://dx.doi.org/10.5772/intechopen.69404

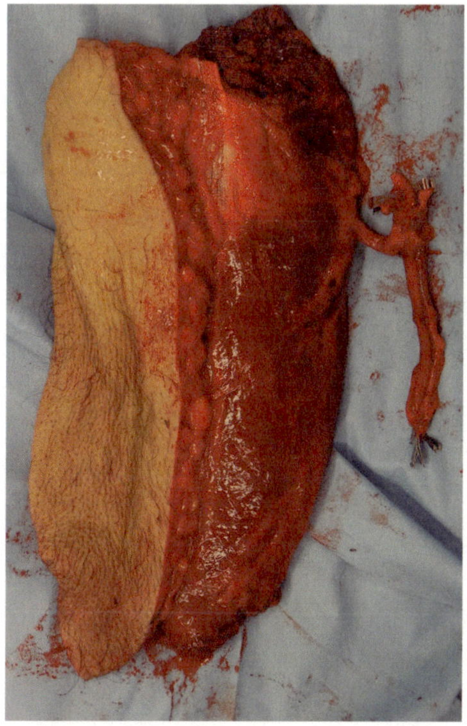

Figure 6. A harvested flow-through ALT flap.

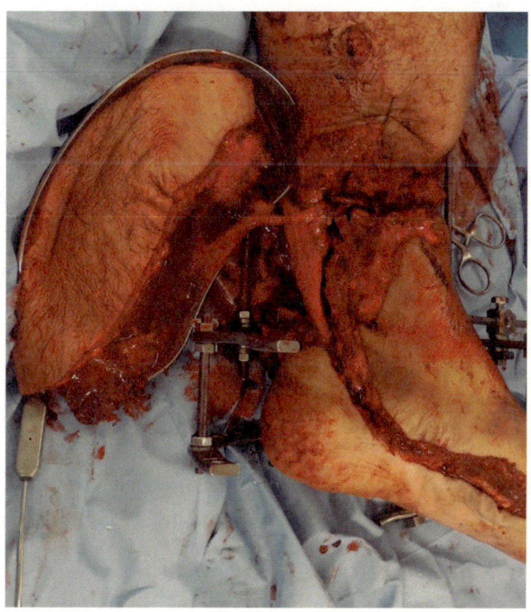

Figure 7. The intra-operative photograph shows the T-portion of the descending branch of the ALT flap interposed within the defect of the posterior tibia artery.

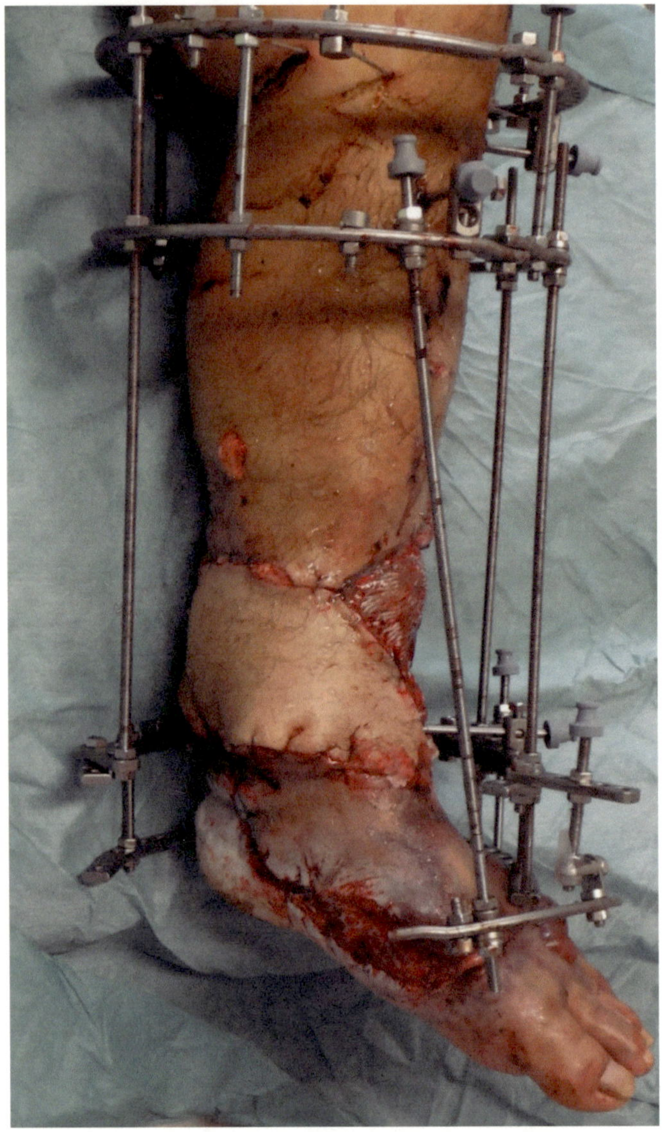

Figure 8. The postoperative photograph shows the resurfacing of all of bone-exposing wound and assumption of circulation to the foot.

a biopsy specimen indicated squamous cell carcinoma. The peripheral side of his lower leg was perfused only by the posterior tibial artery, because both the anterior tibial and peroneal arteries had been interrupted due to a trauma suffered 40 years previously (**Figure 10**).

After the complete removal of the tumor (**Figure 11**), the bone-exposing wound was resurfaced with a free flow-through ALT flap with a 22.0 × 8.0-cm elliptical skin island (**Figure 12**). The T-portion of the descending branch of the lateral circumflex femoral vessel was interposed

http://dx.doi.org/10.5772/intechopen.69404

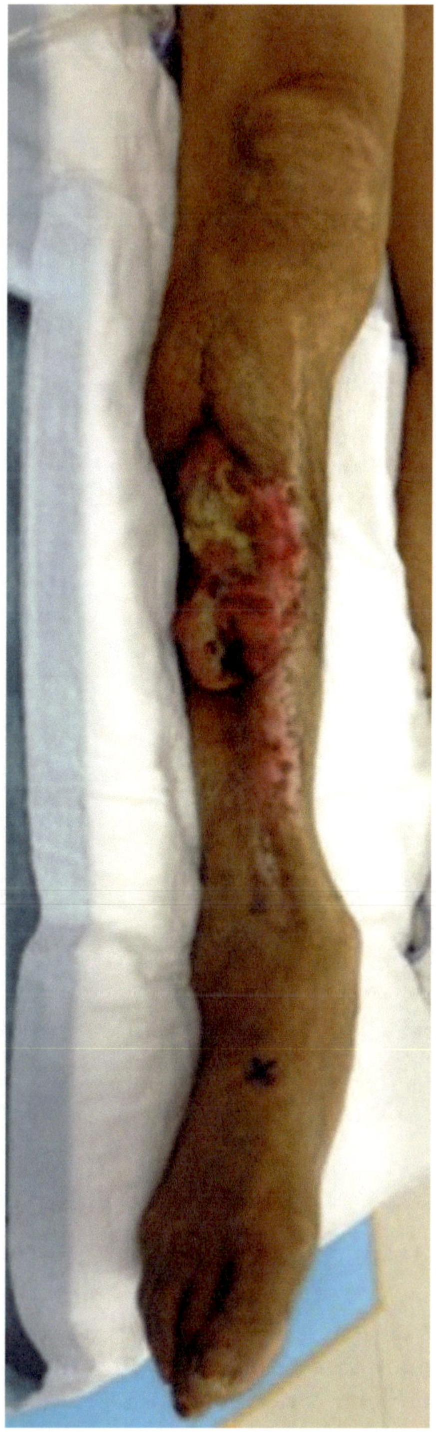

Figure 9. *Case 2.* The photograph shows a chronic right leg ulcer, which developed a fungating wound.

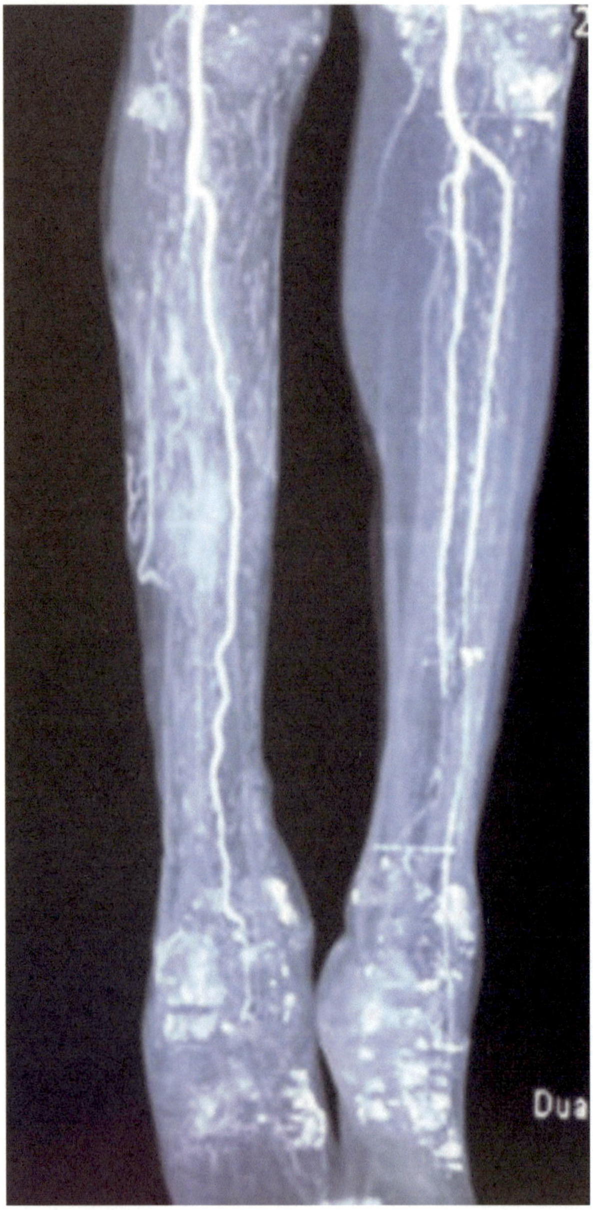

Figure 10. Contrast-enhanced CT revealed that the lower leg was solely being perfused by the posterior tibial artery.

within the divided posterior tibial artery. Two veins were connected to the accompanying posterior tibial veins by end-to-end anastomosis (**Figure 13**). The viability of the skin flaps was favorable without infection or necrosis (**Figure 14**). Contrast-enhanced computed tomography of the reconstructed leg 1 month after surgery demonstrated successful revascularization at the vascular anastomotic sites, which maintained effective circulation of the right foot (**Figure 15**). Six months later, the patient showed a favorable outcome of the lower leg without recurrence (**Figure 16**).

http://dx.doi.org/10.5772/intechopen.69404

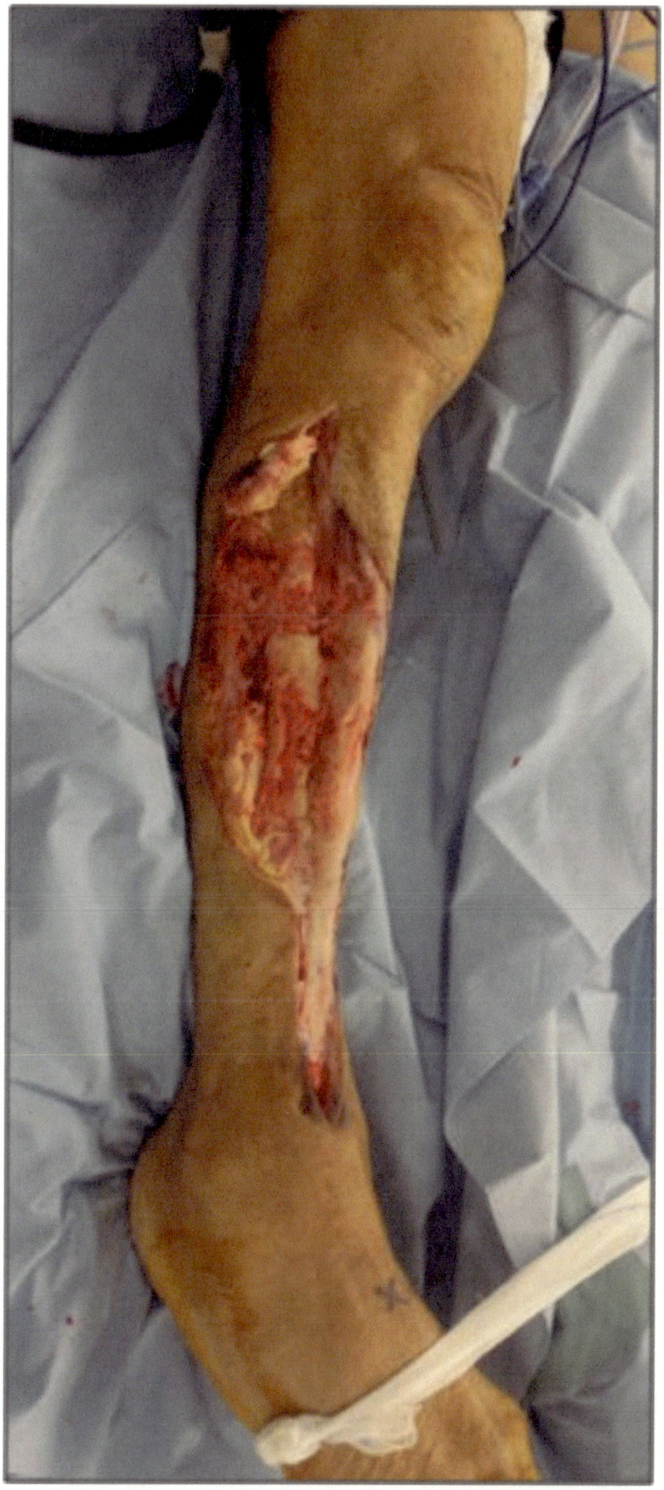

Figure 11. Intraoperative picture after the complete tumor removal showing the large bone-exposing wound.

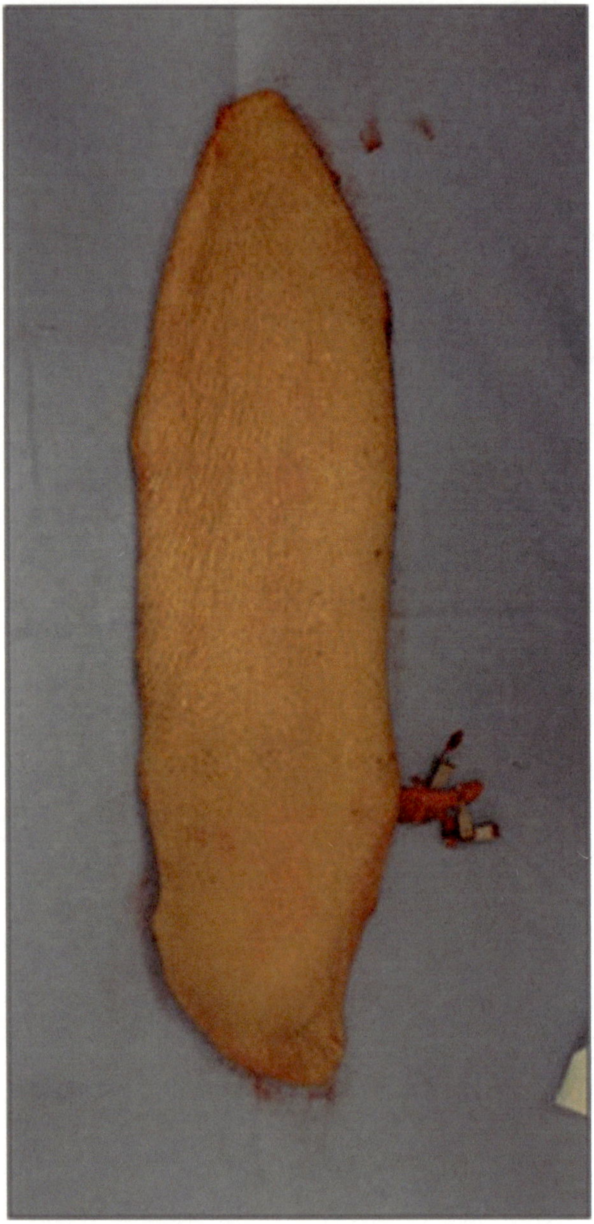

Figure 12. A harvested flow-through ALT flap.

Case 3. A 57-year-old male had developed a diabetic ulcer on the medial malleolus, which had enlarged over a 1-year period. He had non-controlled diabetes mellitus for more than 7 years. There was evidence of peripheral circulatory disturbance. The chronic ulcer reached the fibula and osteomyelitis occurred (**Figure 17**). He underwent debridement that included infected bone. To maintain peripheral circulation, the defect after resection was resurfaced

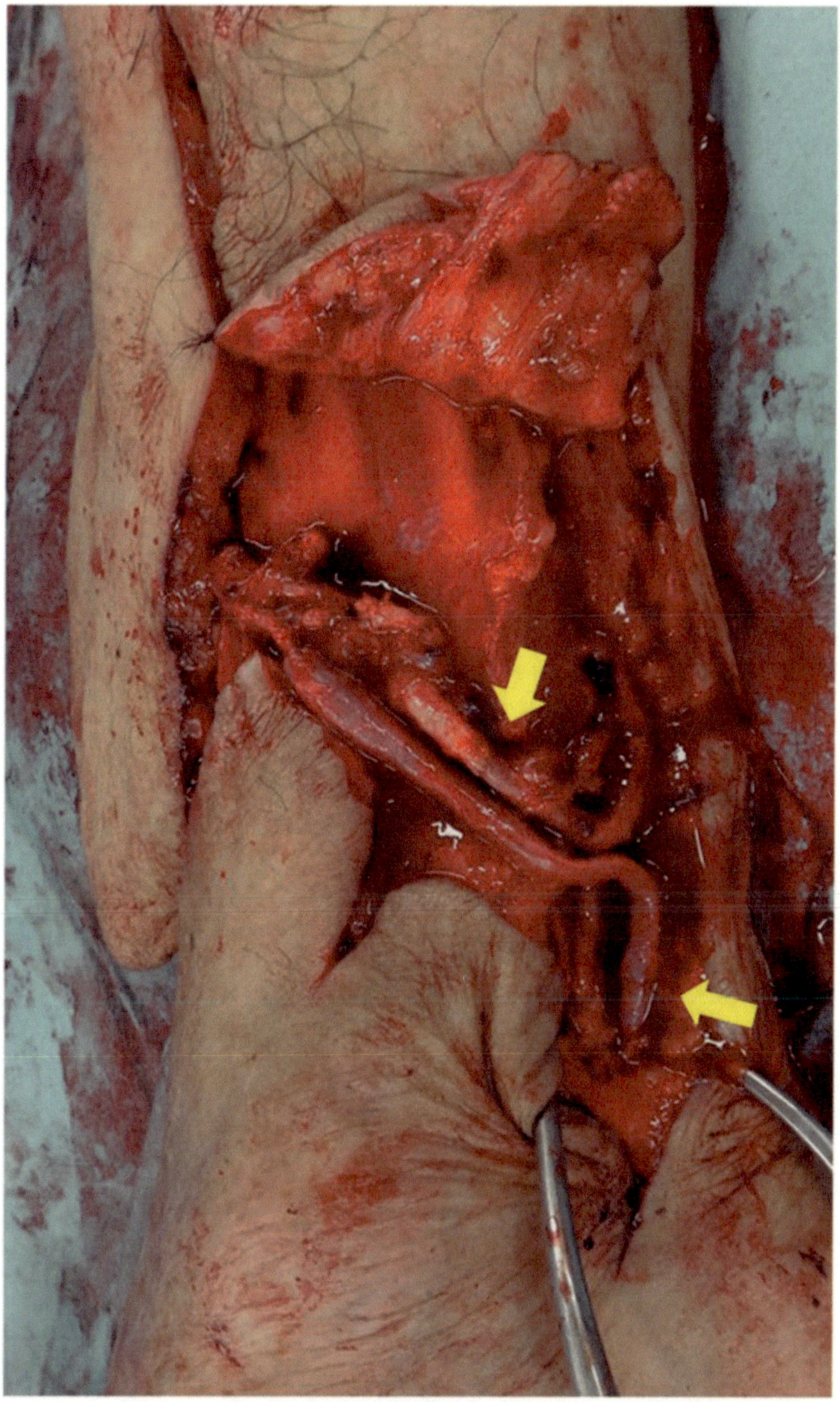

Figure 13. Intraoperative picture showing the T-portion of the descending branch interposed within the divided posterior tibial artery. The arrows indicate the microsurgical anastomosis points.

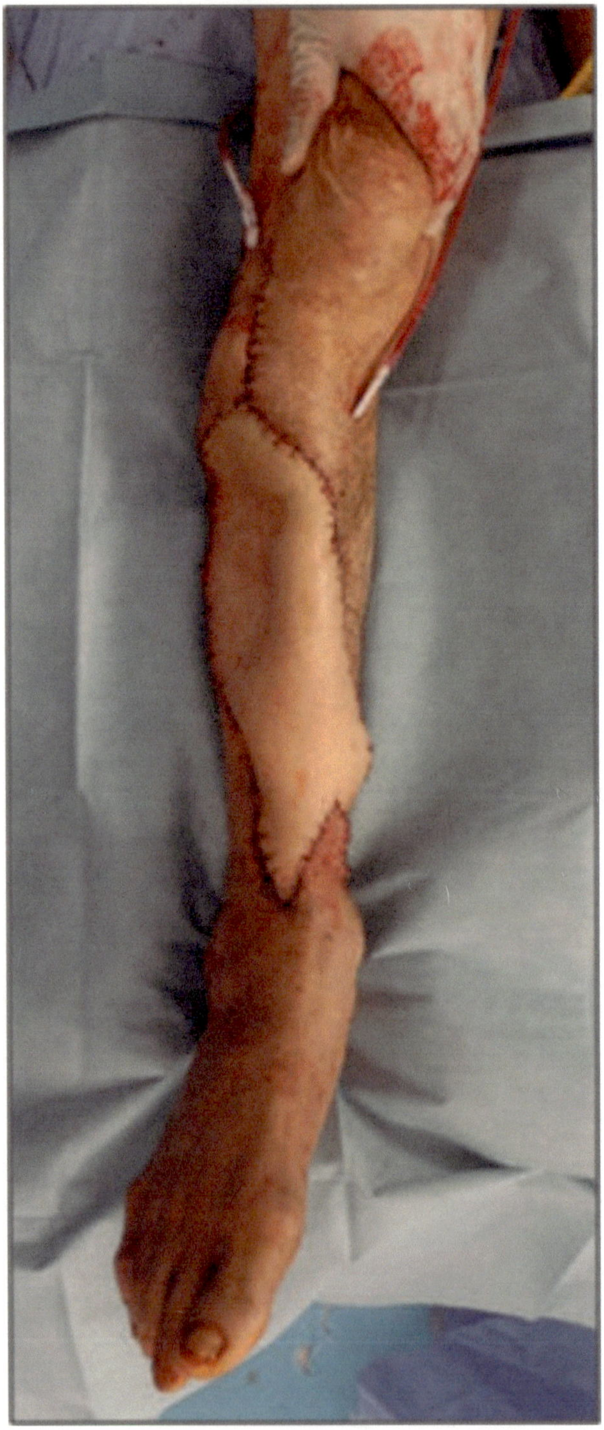

Figure 14. A postoperative photograph showing the resurfacing of all of the bone-exposing wound, and immediate resumption of foot circulation.

http://dx.doi.org/10.5772/intechopen.69404

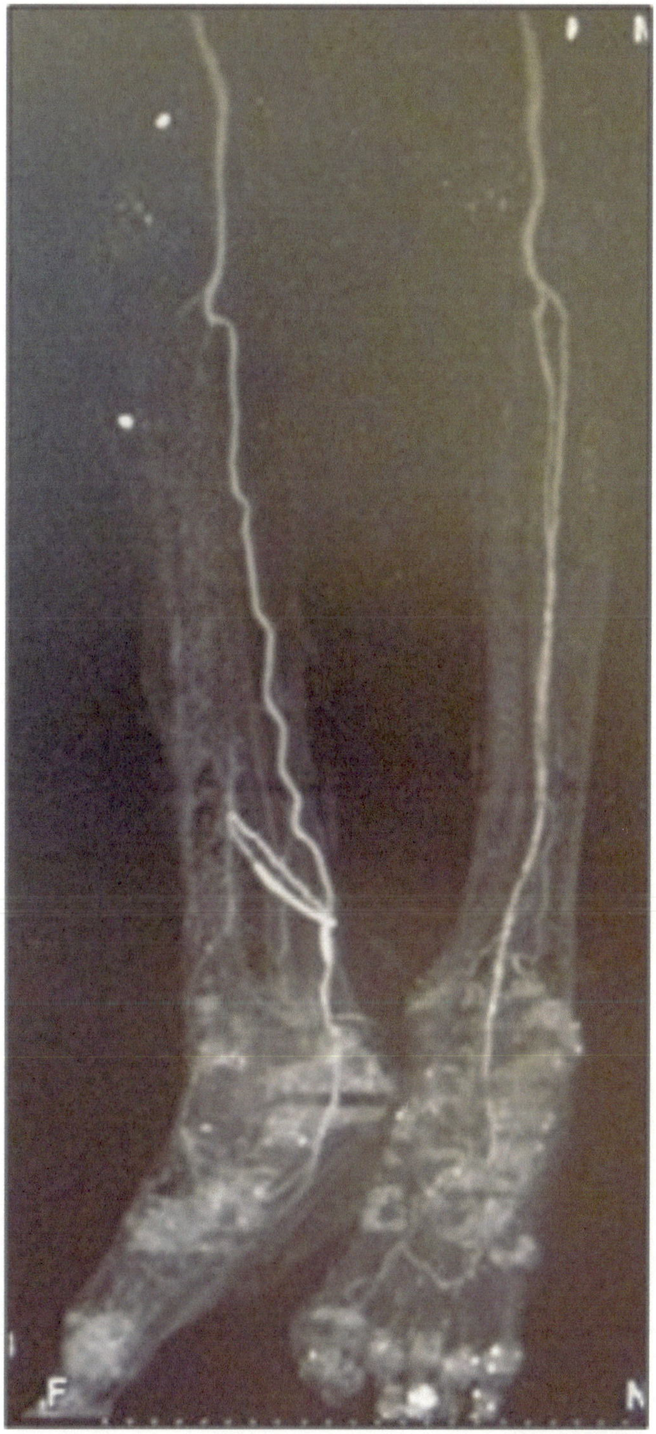

Figure 15. Contrast-enhanced CT demonstrated sufficient circulation of both the transferred flap and right foot.

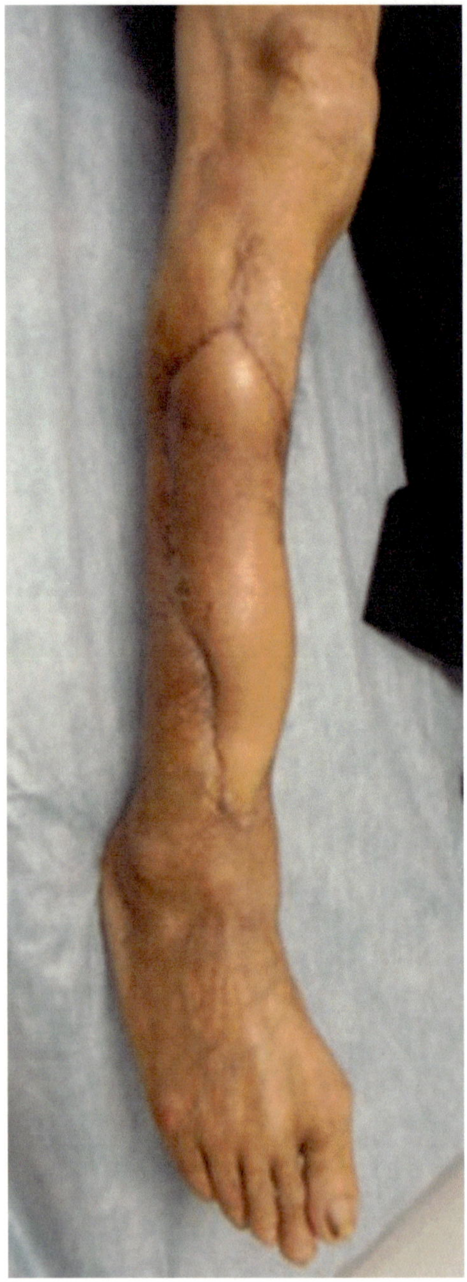

Figure 16. A 6-month postoperative view. The viability of both the leg and flap was favorable, without tumor recurrence.

with a free flow-through ATL fasciocutaneous flap (**Figure 18**). The T-portion of the descending branch was interposed within the posterior tibial vessel. The viability of the skin flaps was favorable without infection or necrosis (**Figure 19**). This flap was thin enough to enable him to wear shoes (**Figure 20**).

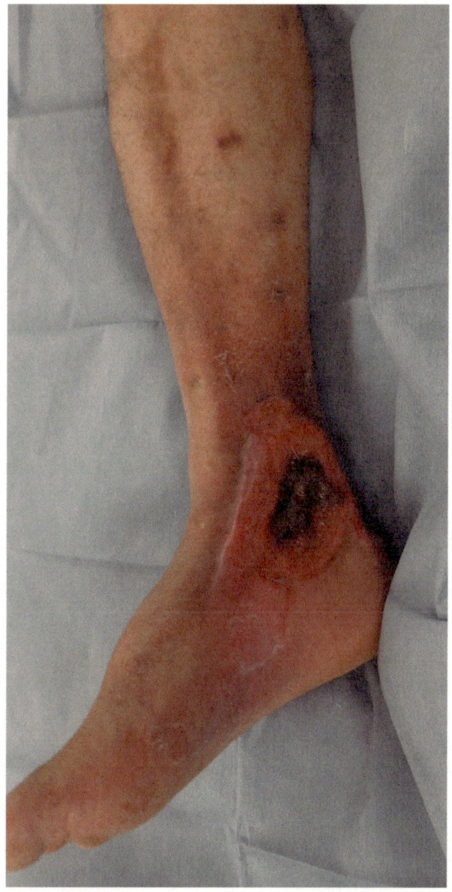

Figure 17. *Case 3*. This photograph shows a diabetic ulcer on the medial malleolus associated with osteomyelitis.

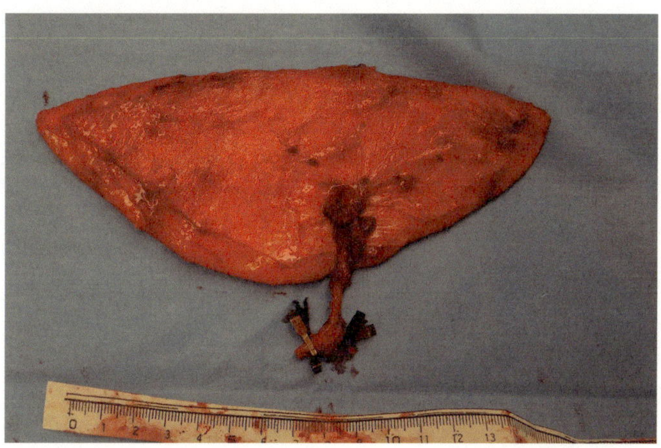

Figure 18. A harvested flow-through ALT fasciocutaneous flap.

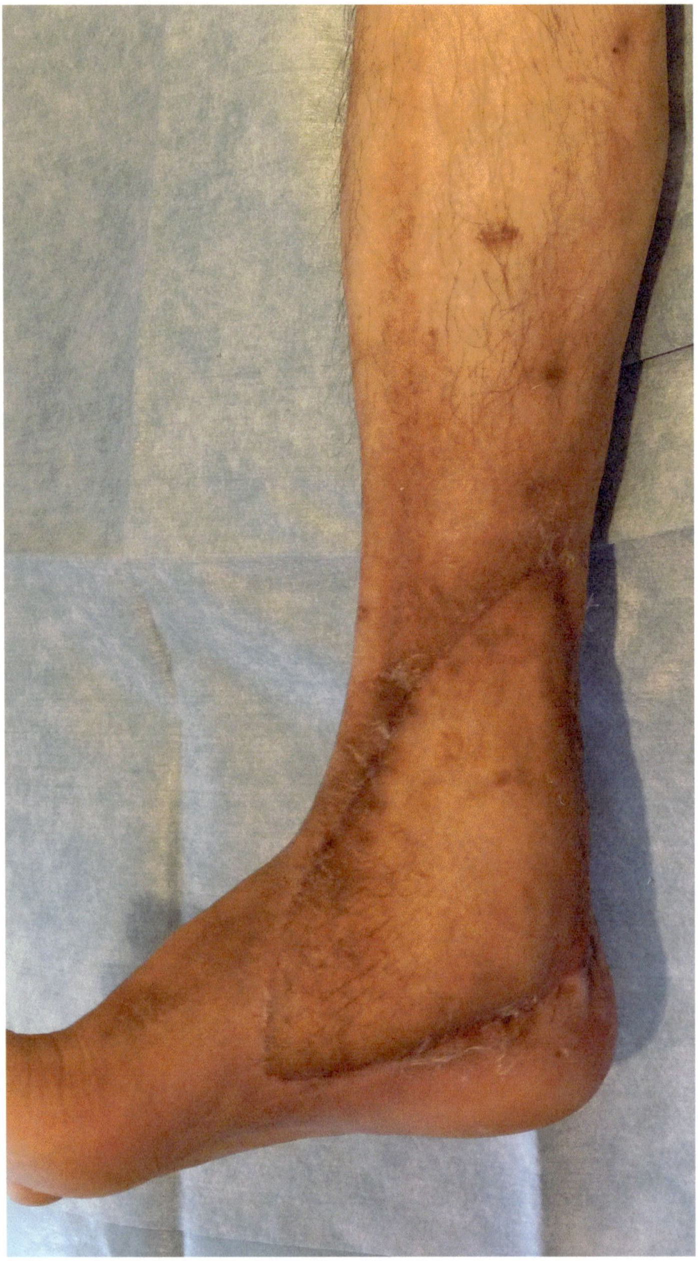

Figure 19. A 6-month post-operative view. The viability of both the leg and flap was favorable, there was no ulcer recurrence.

5.3. Additional blood supply for ischemic flap

As a flow-through flap can supply circulation for distal areas, it may be utilized to improve blood flow to other distally-based ischemic flaps, which show poor circulation [7, 23].

http://dx.doi.org/10.5772/intechopen.69404

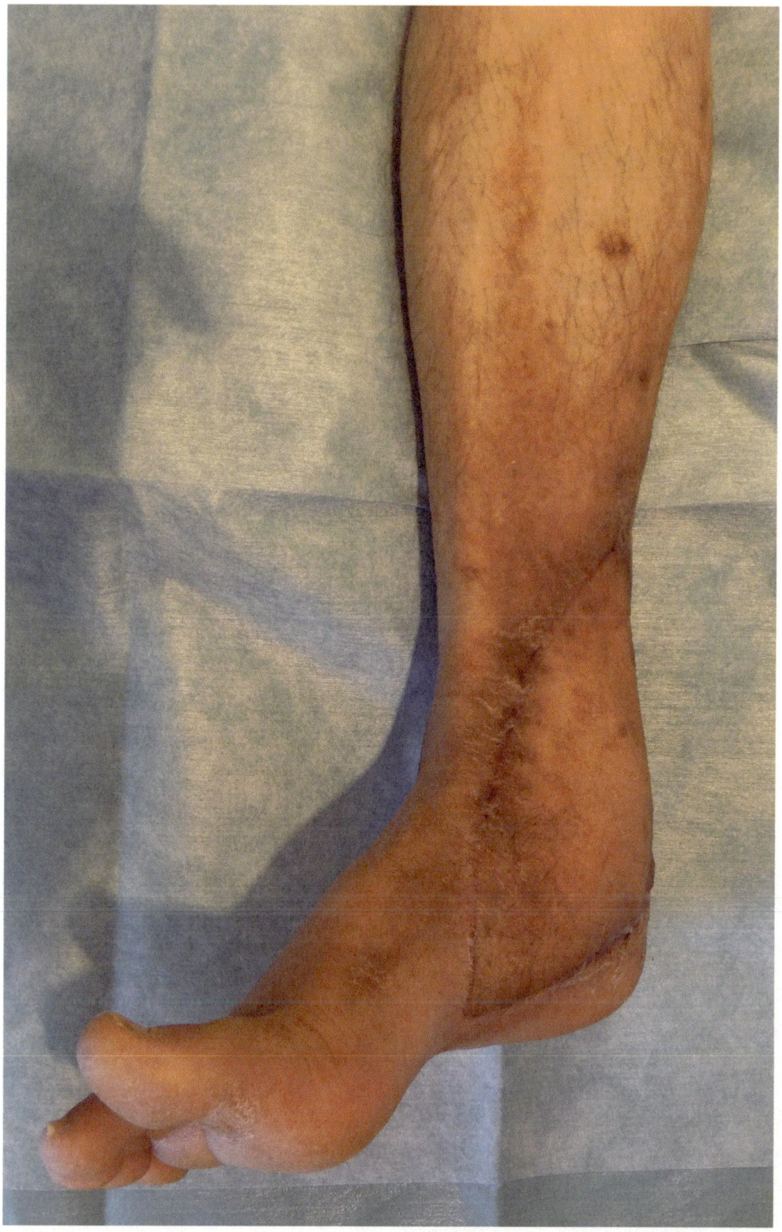

Figure 20. A 6-month post-operative view. The ALT fasciocutaneous flap was thin enough to enable the patient to wear shoes.

Case 4. A 53-year-old man underwent resection of a malignant melanoma presenting at the distolateral plantar weight-bearing region of the right foot (**Figure 21**). The defect after resection of the melanoma was repaired with a reversed island median plantar flap (**Figure 22**). However, the flap became ischemia as the reversed blood flow was insufficient to maintain adequate circulation. Thus, the instep donor defect was covered with a free anterolateral thigh

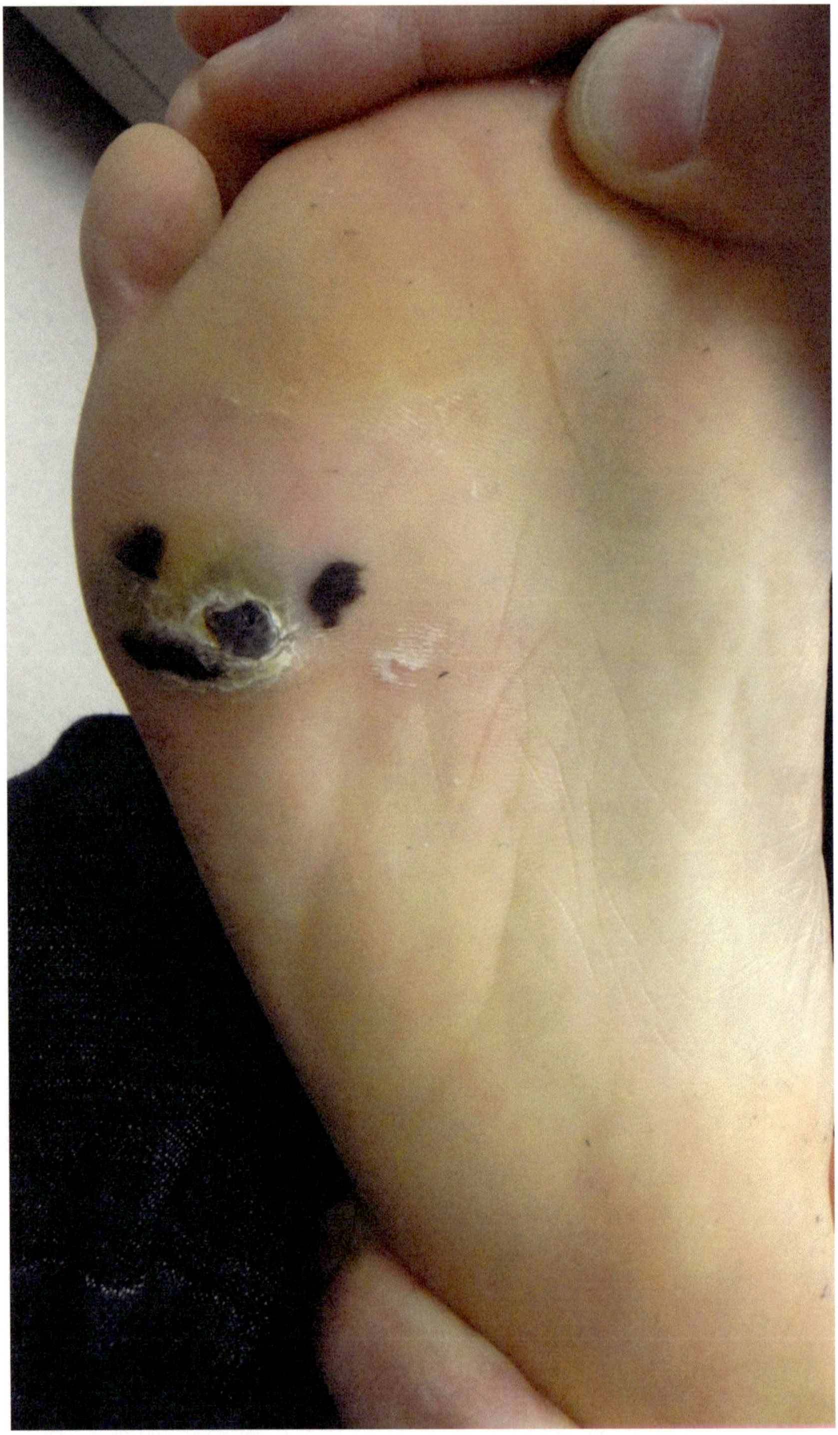

Figure 21. *Case 4*. This photograph shows a malignant melanoma on the distolateral plantar weight-bearing region of the right foot.

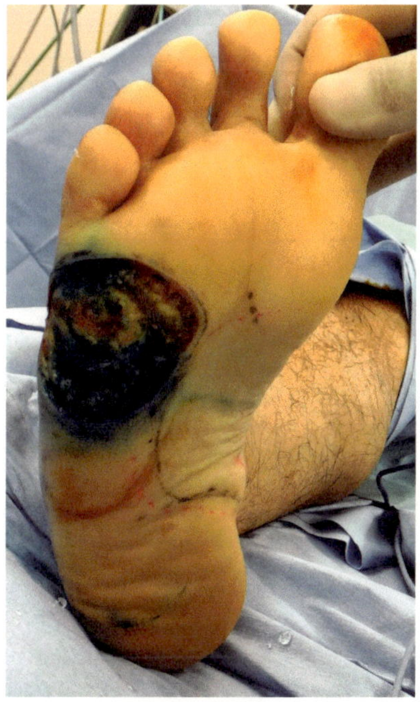

Figure 22. Intraoperative photograph of the wound after complete resection of the tumor.

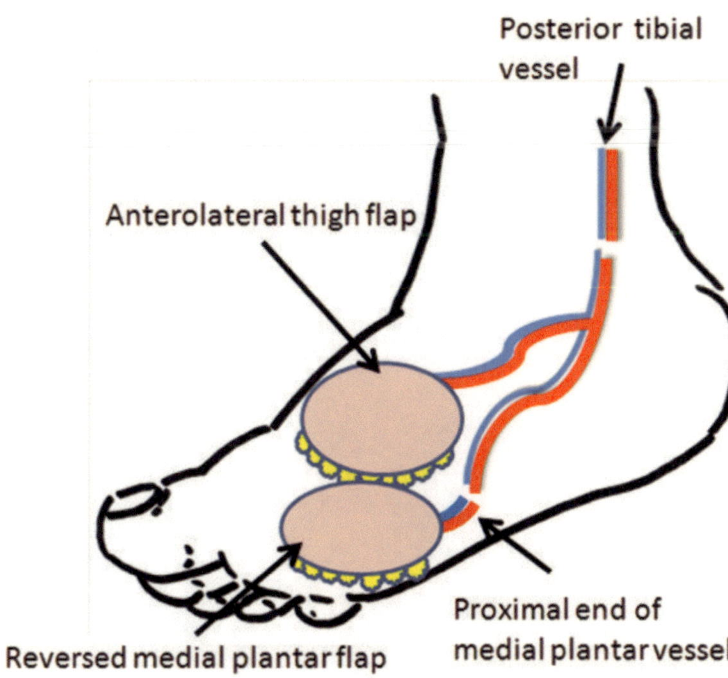

Figure 23. Schematic representation of the instep donor defect coverage with a free flow-through ALT flap.

flap, while the T-portion of the descending branch of the lateral circumflex femoral vessel was interposed within the transected medial plantar vessel providing additional blood supply to the ischemic flap (**Figures 23** and **24**). Consequently, ischemia of the reversed median plantar flap improved, because the interrupted medial plantar vessel resumed normal blood flow (**Figure 25**). The patient could walk without tumor recurrence 1 year after surgery (**Figure 26**).

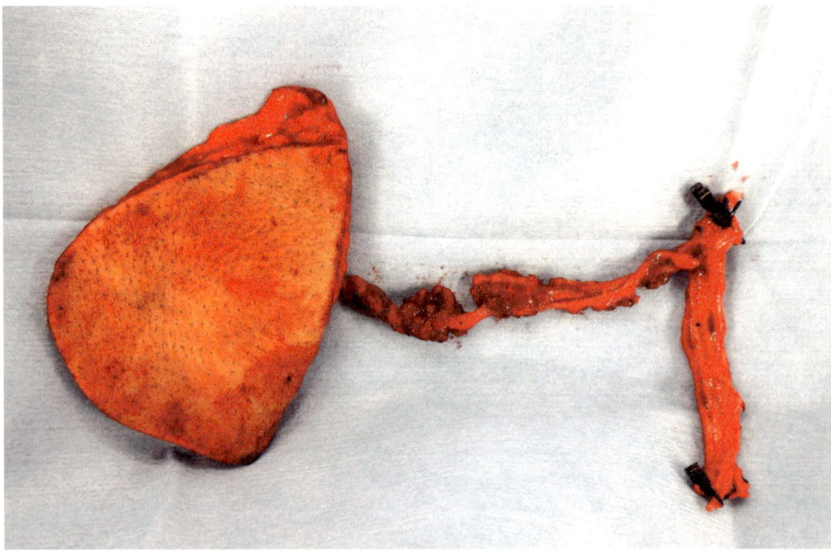

Figure 24. A harvested flow-through ALT flap.

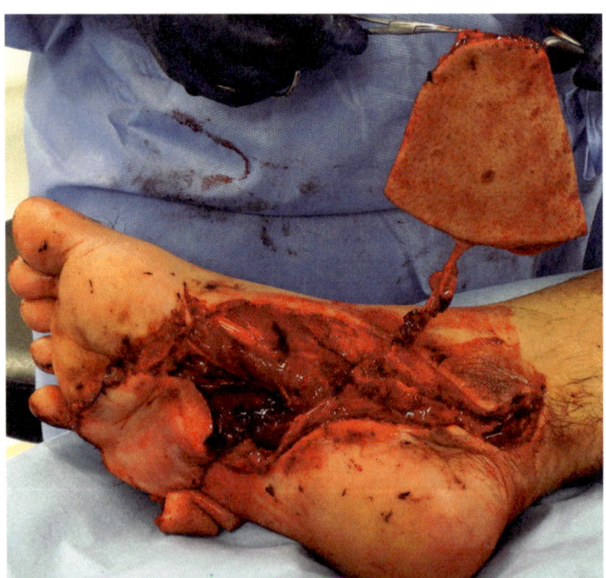

Figure 25. The T-portion of the descending branch was interposed within the transected medial plantar vessel. Subsequently, ischemia of the reversed median plantar flap improved.

http://dx.doi.org/10.5772/intechopen.69404

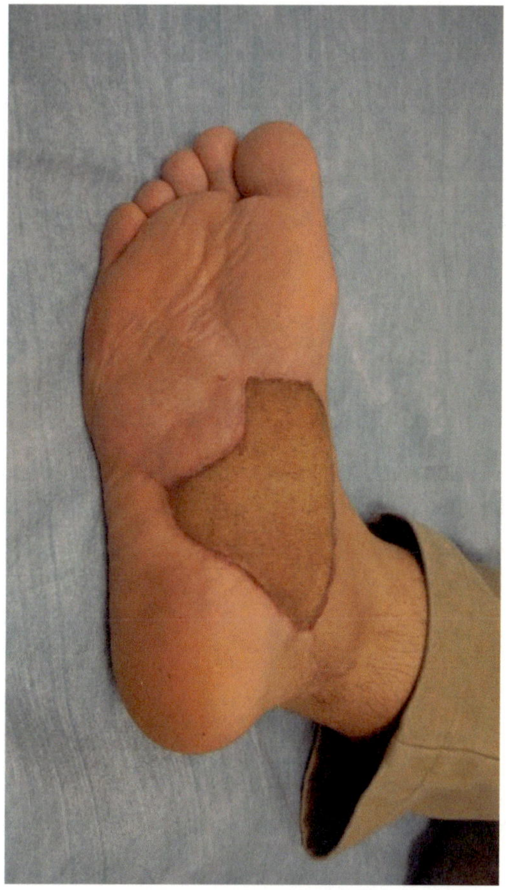

Figure 26. A 12-month postoperative view. The viability of both the leg and flap was favorable; there was no tumor recurrence.

6. Discussion

Reconstruction of soft tissue defects in areas of the extremities with no or impaired circulation is one of the most difficult challenges. Surgeons must reconstruct the defect as well as maintain the peripheral circulation, or patients will lose their limbs. A flow-through flap may be utilized in an effort to reconstruct the vasculature as well as provide soft tissue coverage [24].

The author believes that this flap is useful not only for establishing arterial blood supply to the peripheral tissue, but also for preserving venous return, especially in legs with venous stasis. This is particularly so, because it does not sacrifice the valuable deep venous return system. Furthermore, several investigators have reported that flow-through arterial anastomosis leads to a higher patency rate than conventional end-to-end and end-to-side arterial anastomosis, and even promoted more favorable blood flow through the anastomotic site [25, 26].

7. Conclusion

The principal advantage of the flow-through flap is that it allows a single-stage composite reconstruction of both soft tissue and vascular defects, making it particularly useful in the reconstruction of ischemic extremities and defects resulting from oncologic ablations.

Author details

Masaki Fujioka

Address all correspondence to: mfujioka@nagasaki-mc.com

Department of Plastic and Reconstructive Surgery, Clinical Research Center, National Hospital Organization Nagasaki Medical Center, Ohmura City, Japan

References

[1] Clymer MA, Burkey BB. Other flaps for head and neck use: Temporoparietal fascial free flap, lateral arm free flap, omental free flap. Facial Plastic Surgery. 1996;**12**(1):81-89. DOI:10.1055/s-2008-1064498

[2] Shindo ML, Sullivan MJ. Soft-tissue microvascular free flaps. Otolaryngologic Clinics of North America. 1994;**27**(1):1731-1794

[3] Coleman JJ 3rd. Reconstruction of the pharynx and cervical esophagus. Seminars in Surgical Oncology. 1995;**11**(3):208-220

[4] Baker SR. Microvascular free flaps in soft-tissue augmentation of the head and neck. Archives of Otolaryngology--Head & Neck Surgery. 1986;**112**(7):733-737

[5] Saint-Cyr M, Langstein HN. Reconstruction of the hand and upper extremity after tumor resection. Journal of Surgical Oncology. 2006;**94**:490-503. DOI:10.1002/jso.20486

[6] Fujioka M, Hayashida K, Murakami C. Emergent free flow-through anterolateral thigh flaps for Gustilo-Anderson III fracture of the upper extremity. Journal of Emergencies, Trauma and Shock. 2014;**7**(1):53-55. DOI: 10.4103/0974-2700.125642

[7] Fujioka M, Hayashida K, Senju C. Reconstruction of lateral forefoot using reversed medial plantar flap with free anterolateral thigh flap. Journal of Foot and Ankle Surgery. 2014;**53**:324-327. DOI: 10.1053/j.jfas.2013.12.012

[8] Costa H, Cunha C, Conde A, Barsdley A, McGrouther DA. The flow-through free flap in replantation surgery: A new concept. European Journal of Plastic Surgery. 1997;**20**(4)181-185. DOI: 10.1007/BF01152186

[9] Soutar DS, Scheker LR, Tanner NS, McGregor IA. The radial forearm flap: A versatile method for intra-oral reconstruction. British Journal of Plastic Surgery. 1983;**36**(1):1-8

[10] Koshima I, Fujitsu M, Ushio S, Sugiyama N, Yamashita S. Flow-through anterior thigh flaps with a short pedicle for reconstruction of lower leg and foot defects. Plastic and Reconstructive Surgery. 2005;**115**(1):155-162. DOI:10.1055/s-2008-1040770

[11] Miyamoto S, Kayano S, Umezawa H, Fujiki M, Sakuraba M. Flow-through fibula flap using soleus branch as distal runoff:. A case report. Microsurgery. 2013;**33**(1):606-602. DOI:10.1002/micr.22043

[12] Garvey PB, Clemens MW, Rhines LD, Sacks JM. Vertical rectus abdominis musculo-cutaneous flow-through flap to a free fibula flap for total sacrectomy reconstruction. Microsurgery. 2013;**33**(1):32-38. DOI: 10.1002/micr.21990

[13] Rowsell AR, Davies DM, Eisenberg N, Taylor GI. The anatomy of the subscapular-thoracodorsal arterial system: study of 100 cadaver dissections. British Journal of Plastic Surgery. 1984;**37**:574-576

[14] Xu DC, Zhong SZ, Kong JM, Wang GY, Liu MZ, Luo LS, Gao JH. Applied anatomy of the anterolateral femoral flap. Plastic and Reconstructive Surgery. 1988;**82**:305-310

[15] Ceulemans P, Hofer SO. Flow-through anterolateral thigh flap for a free osteocutaneous fibula flap in secondary composite mandible reconstruction. British Journal of Plastic Surgery. 2004;**57**(4):358-361. DOI:10.1016/j.bjps.2004.02.013

[16] Ao M, Nagase Y, Mae O, Namba Y. Reconstruction of posttraumatic defects of the foot by flow-through anterolateral or anteromedial thigh flaps with preservation of posterior tibial vessels. Annals of Plastic Surgery. 1997;**38**:598-603

[17] Wong CH, Wei FC. Anterolateral thigh flap. Head and Neck. 2010;**32**(4):529-540. DOI: 10.1002/hed.21204. DOI:10.1002/hed.21204

[18] Wei FC, Jain V, Celik N, Chen HC, Chuang DC, Lin CH. Have we found an ideal soft-tissue flap? An experience with 672 anterolateral thigh flaps. Plastic and Reconstructive Surgery. 2002;**109**:2219-2226

[19] Gokhan M, Ulusal AE, Atik A, Sargin S, Ulusal B, Sukru Sahin M. Descending branch of the lateral circumflex femoral artery as a recipient vessel for vascularized fibular grafts: Clinical case series. Microsurgery. 2014;**34**(8):633-637. DOI: 10.1002/micr.22299

[20] Haffey TM, Lamarre ED, Fritz MA. Auto flow-through technique for anterolateral Thigh Flaps. JAMA Facial Plastic Surgery. 2014;**16**(2):147-150. DOI:10.1001/jamafacial.2013.2263

[21] Fujioka M, Hayashida K, Murakami C. Artificial dermis is not effective for resurfacing bone-exposing wounds of Gustilo-Anderson III fracture. Journal of Plastic, Reconstructive & Aesthetic Surgery. 2013;**66**(4):e119-121. DOI: 10.1016/j.bjps.2012.12.005

[22] Kells AF, Broyles JM, Simoa AF, Lewis VO, Sacks JM. Anterolateral thigh flow-through flap in hand salvage. Eplasty. 2013;**13**:e19

[23] Oberlin C, Accioli de Vasconcellos Z, Touam C. Medial plantar flap based distally on the lateral plantar artery to cover a forefoot skin defect. Plastic and Reconstructive Surgery. 2000;**106**:874-877

[24] Hidalgo DA. Aesthetic improvements in free-flap mandible reconstruction. Plastic and Reconstructive Surgery. 1991;**88**:574-585

[25] Kim JT, Kim CY, Kim YH. T-anastomosis in microsurgical free flap reconstruction: An overview of clinical applications. Journal of Plastic, Reconstructive & Aesthetic Surgery. 2008;**61**:1157-1163. DOI:10.1016/j.bjps.2008.03.048

[26] Miyamoto S, Okazaki M, Ohura N, Shiraishi T, Takushima A, Harii K. Comparative study of different combinations of microvascular anastomoses in a rat model: end-to-end, end-to-side, and flow-through anastomosis. Plastic and Reconstructive Surgery. 2008;**122**:449-455. DOI:10.1097/PRS.0b013e31817d62c5

Chapter 5

Emergent or Early Flap Resurfacing Is Required for Bone-Exposing Wounds of Gustilo-Anderson IIIB and IIIC Fractures

Masaki Fujioka

Additional information is available at the end of the chapter

http://dx.doi.org/10.5772/intechopen.70147

Abstract

Background: The wound treatment has progressed owing to the development of new medicine, instruments. Following these trends, can the bone-exposing wounds of severe open fractures be resurfaced without using flaps but only skin grafting? We evaluated a new medicine and instrument, for the resurfacing of bone-exposing complex wounds of Gustilo-Anderson IIIB and C fractures. Patients and methods: Patients with Gustilo-Anderson IIIB (five cases) and C (two cases) open fractures who underwent open reduction and external fixation were evaluated. Bone-exposing wounds were resurfaced with artificial dermis, and basic fibroblast growth factor was sprayed. We investigated the course and outcome. Result: In all of seven cases, abundant granulation tissue did not develop on the bone-exposing wound surface during 2–5 weeks, and 4 patients developed osteomyelitis. Subsequently, all cases required flap surgery to resurface the wound. All patients could walk; however, required a longer period for the complete union of bones. Conclusion: This study showed that it was impossible to prepare a favorable wound bed on the bone when the fracture was severe. Thus, early flap surgery was a recommendable resurfacing option. Furthermore, emergent bone resurfacing with flap, while performing rigid bone fixation with an internal fixation plate, was an ideal procedure.

Keywords: emergent reconstruction, free flow-through flap, anterolateral thigh flap, Gustilo-Anderson IIIB and C fractures, vascular repair

1. Introduction

Gustilo-Anderson type III fracture is defined as an open fracture with extensive soft-tissue laceration, damage, or loss or an open segmental fracture, and type IIIB as a severe that open fracture with extensive soft-tissue loss. The severest open fracture is called type IIIC; it is associated with an arterial injury requiring immediate repair [1]. The resurfacing of bone-exposing complex wounds of this type of fracture remains challenging. Previous conventional wound management involved leaving wounds open after debridement; this might have been because antibiotics and surgical debridement did not prevail, and soft-tissue reconstructive techniques had not been developed [2–5].

Recent technological advances of wound management have made the healing of complex chronic wounds earlier and easier [6, 7]. The development of new medicines, instruments, and techniques, including artificial dermis, angiogenic cytokines, and negative pressure wound treatment device, has allowed bone-exposing wounds to heal more quickly [8, 9]. Among these, artificial dermis is beneficial for the resurfacing of wounds with exposed tendons or bone. Its unique granular regeneration promoting characteristic even on bare bone may allow resurfacing with a free skin graft. Thus, it may replace flap surgery for the treatment of several bone-exposing wounds including deep burns, postabrasion of neoplasms, and skin defects due to trauma (**Figures 1–3**) [10, 11].

It is generally felt difficult to prepare a favorable wound bed on the bone when the open fracture is too severe and complex, such as those classified as Gustilo-Anderson IIIB and C. This work is divided into three sections. In the first section, we present and discuss the outcome of resurfacing Gustilo-Anderson IIIB and C bone-exposing wounds, subjected to late treatment using artificial dermis. In the second section, we describe and discuss cases of successful

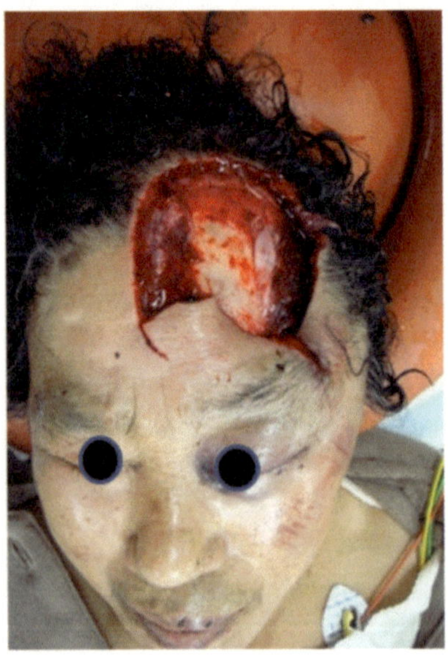

Figure 1. Case 1. This picture shows a forehead injury with a skin defect exposing frontal bone. Artificial dermis was applied to the wound.

http://dx.doi.org/10.5772/intechopen.70147

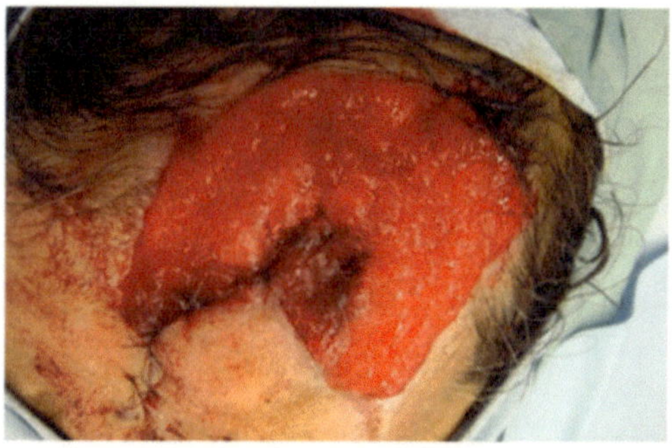

Figure 2. The wound was covered with granulation tissue 4 weeks after injury; thus, a full-thickness skin graft could be performed.

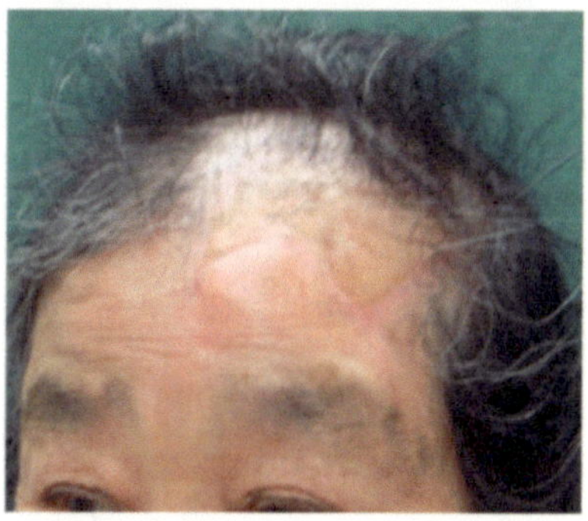

Figure 3. Photograph at 3 months postinjury showing the resurfacing of all of the bone-exposing wound.

salvage and reconstruction of Gustilo-Anderson IIIC extremity fractures, highlighting the advantage of emergent free flow-through flap resurfacing. In the third section, we introduce and discuss the "fix and flap" concept, a new radical concept for the treatment of severe open fractures.

2. Disadvantages of conventional late resurfacing for Gustilo-Anderson IIIB and C bone-exposing wounds

Conventional options to treat Gustilo-Anderson IIIB and C bone-exposing injuries are primary surgery including debridement and cleansing, vascular repair, bone reduction/external fixation, and secondary wound resurfacing surgery by skin graft and pedicle or free flap transfer (**Figures 4–8**) [12–14]. Ideally, all procedure should be performed immediately; however, the resurfacing of wound tends to be performed late, because of concerns over the development of wound infection or shortage of surgical staff for emergent surgery. In these cases,

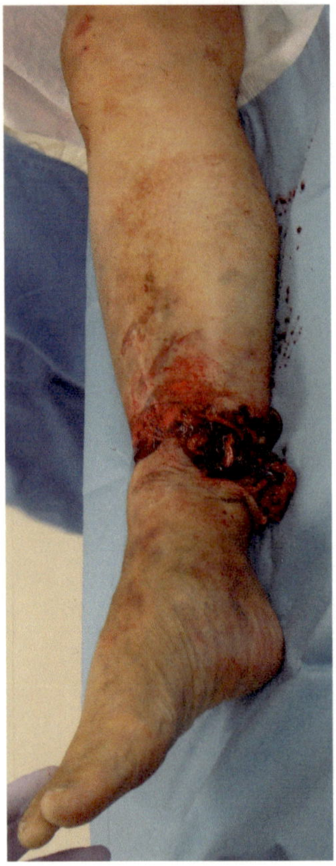

Figure 4. Case 2. Conventional treatment of Gustilo-Anderson IIIC fracture. The patient sustained an open fracture to the right leg.

pending secondary surgery, the wound is dressed temporarily with wet gauze, several wound dressing materials, or artificial dermis. Our practice has been to apply artificial dermis on the bone, expecting granulation. In this section, we present the outcome of resurfacing Gustilo-Anderson IIIB and C wounds, which had been treated with artificial dermis.

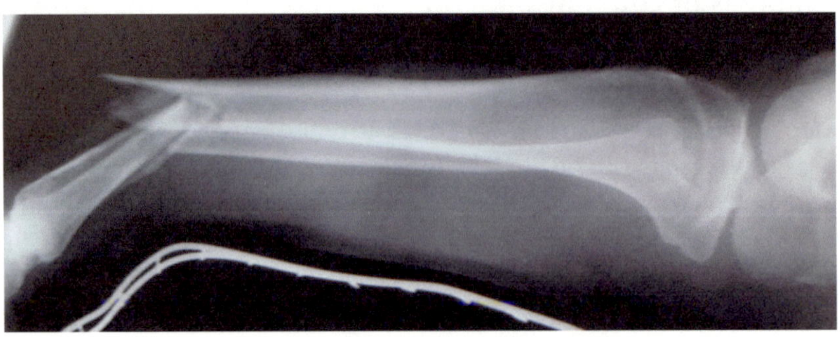

Figure 5. The X-ray image shows both tibia and fibula fractures.

http://dx.doi.org/10.5772/intechopen.70147

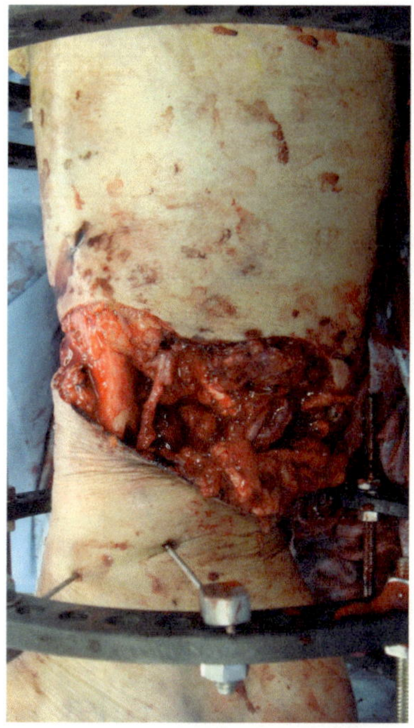

Figure 6. After reduction and external fixation, the posterior tibial artery was repaired with an interposition of vein graft. The wound was covered temporarily with artificial dermis.

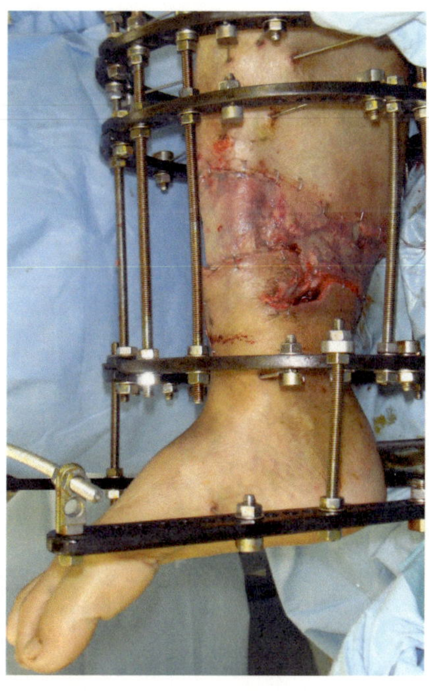

Figure 7. Three weeks later, the wound was resurfaced by local skin flap and free skin graft.

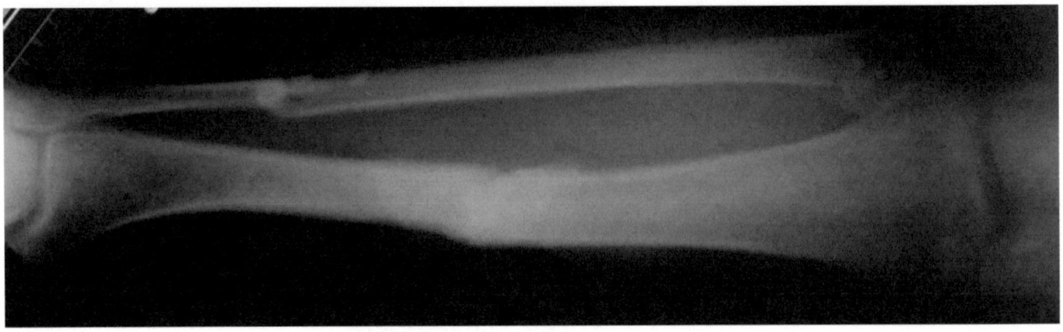

Figure 8. The X-ray image months later shows favorable bone union.

3. Patients and method

A total of seven patients with Gustilo-Anderson III B (five cases) and C (two cases) open fracture were treated in the National Organization Nagasaki Medical Center in 2011 and 2012 (**Table 1**). All patients underwent open reduction and Ilizarov external fixation. Artificial dermis (TerudermisR, Orimpas-Terumo Co., Ltd., Tokyo, Japan) and ointment-impregnated gauze were applied to the wounds.

	Age sex	Site of open fracture	Gustilo-Anderson classification	Complication	Surgical resurfacing (postinjury period, week)	Additional surgery	Prognosis/ external fixation period
1	74 M	Rt. tibia and fibula	IIIC (PTA reconstruction)	–	Local flap (5 W)	–	Walk/4 months
2	58 M	Rt. tibia and fibula	IIIB	–	Local flap (3 W)	–	Walk/6 months
3	32 M	Rt. tibia and fibula	IIIB	Osteomyelitis	Sequestration (2 W), local flap (5 W)	Sequestrectomy	Walk/13 months
4	68 M	Rt. tibia and fibula	IIIB	Osteomyelitis	Local flap (W)	Bone grafting	Walk/11 months
5	44 M	Rt. tibia and fibula	IIIB	Osteomyelitis	Sequestration, local flap (2 W)	Sequestrectomy	Walk/18 months
6	56 M	Rt. tibia	IIIC (PTA reconstruction)	Osteomyelitis	Local flap (4 W)	–	Walk/11 months
7	74 M	Rt. tibia and fibula	IIIB	–	Local flap (W)	–	Walk/10 months

PTA: Posterior tibial artery, FSG: Free skin grafting

Table 1. Cases of patients with Gustilo-Anderson IIIB and C open fracture who were treated with artificial dermis.

4. Results

In all of the seven cases, abundant granulation tissue did not develop on the bone-exposing wound surface during 2–5 weeks after applying the artificial dermis to the bone. Four patients developed osteomyelitis and required continuous irrigation. Among them, two underwent sequestrectomy (**Figures 9–12**). Subsequently, all cases required local flap transfer to resurface the bone-exposing wound (**Figures 13–16**). One patient developed malunion and required bone grafting. Patients suffering from complications required a longer period for the complete union of bones, a fact which prolonged the fixation period (11–18 months). Finally, all patients could walk after removal of the external fixation (**Figures 17** and **18**).

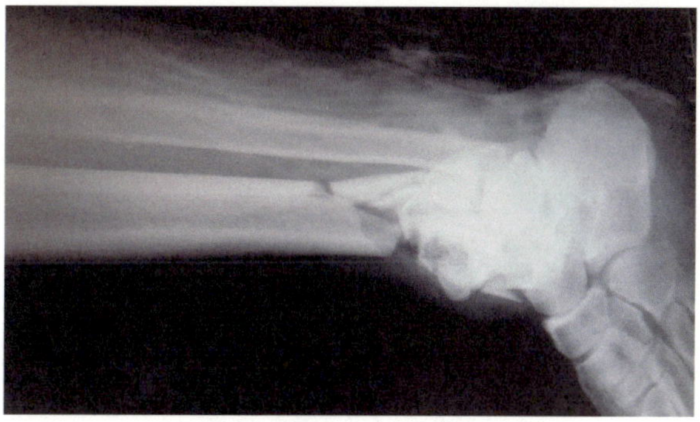

Figure 9. Case 3. The unpleasant course of Gustilo-Anderson IIIB fracture treated with conventional late wound resurfacing. The patient sustained an open fracture to the right leg.

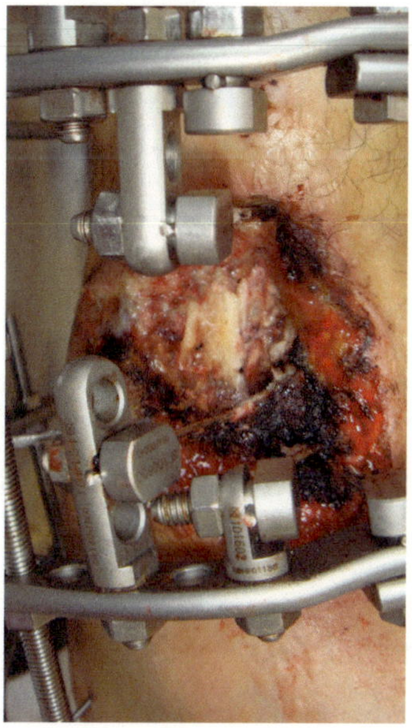

Figure 10. After reduction and external fixation, the wound was covered temporarily with artificial dermis. The picture shows osteomyelitis 2 weeks later.

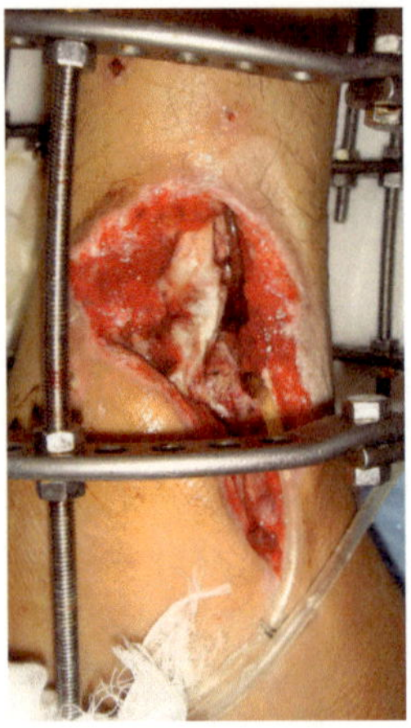

Figure 11. After sequestrectomy and continuous wound irrigation, the wound was cleansed. Next, the wound was resurfaced by local skin flap and free skin graft 3 weeks later.

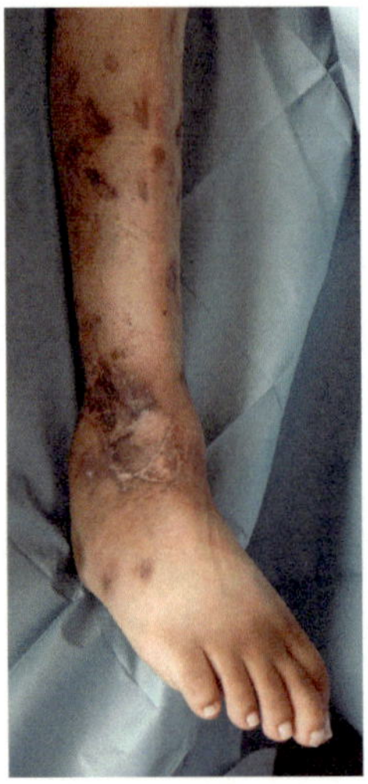

Figure 12. The picture shows the appearance of the injured leg. The patient took 6 months to walk.

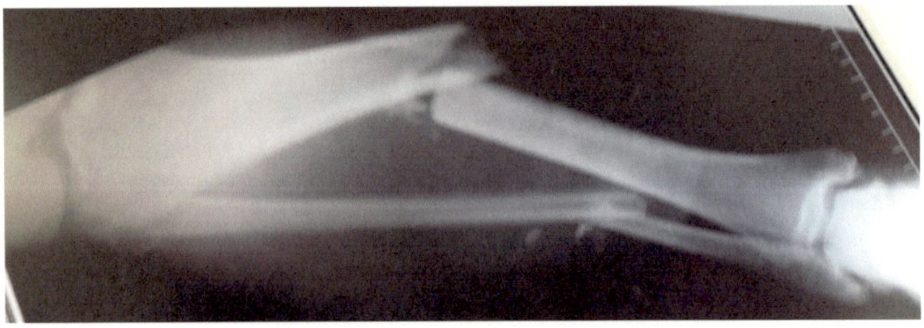

Figure 13. Case 4. The patient sustained a Gustilo-Anderson IIIB open fracture to both tibia and fibula.

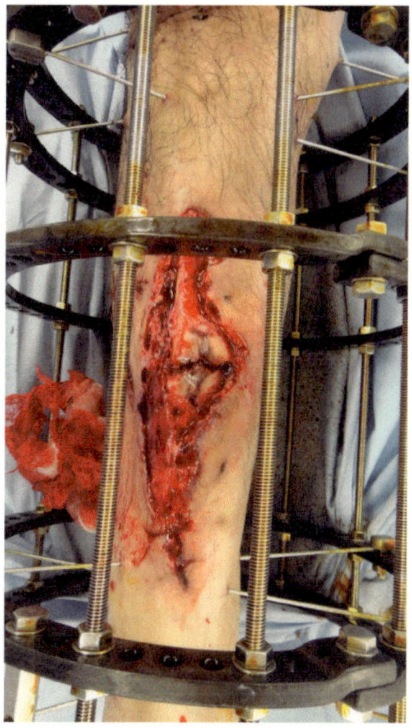

Figure 14. The wound was covered temporarily with artificial dermis. The picture shows absence of granulation growth on the bone 3 weeks later.

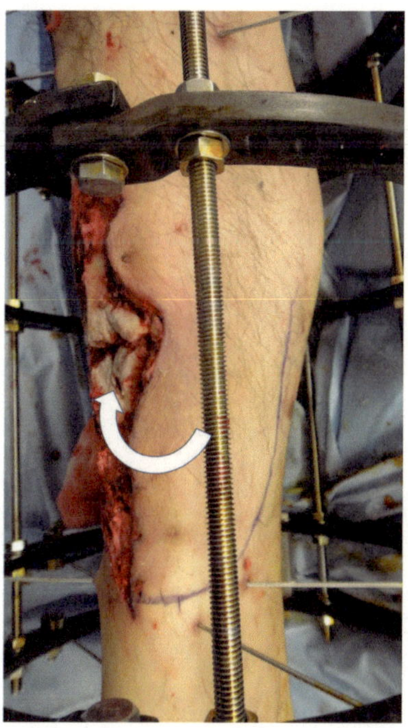

Figure 15. A local skin flap and a free skin were planned to resurface the wound. The picture shows the design of the flap.

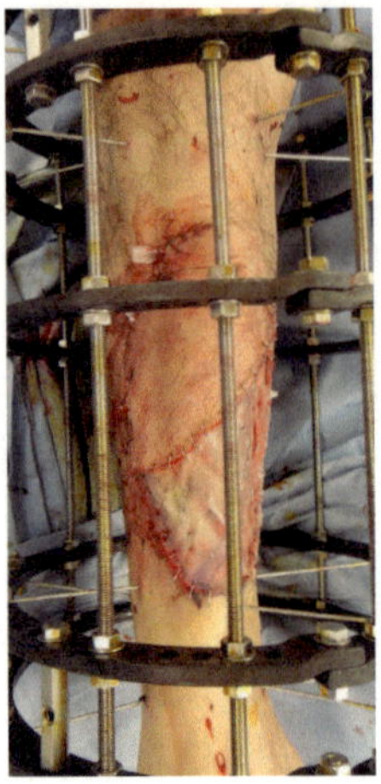

Figure 16. The picture shows a postoperative view. The bone-exposed wound was covered with flap, the remaining wound received a free skin graft.

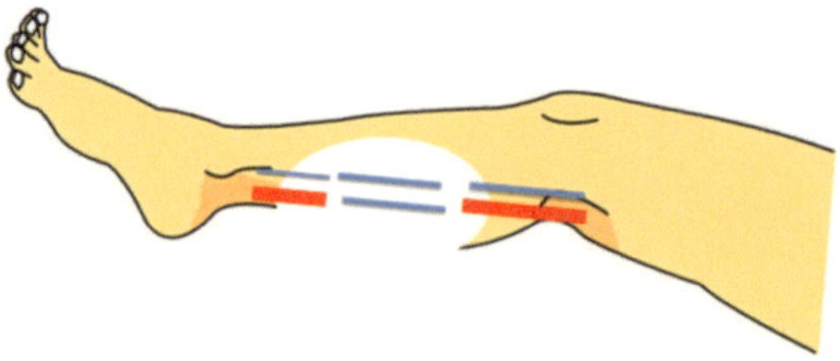

Figure 17. Schematic representation of the conventional procedure of vascular repair for Gustilo-Anderson IIIC fracture. This method requires additional flap surgery for wound coverage.

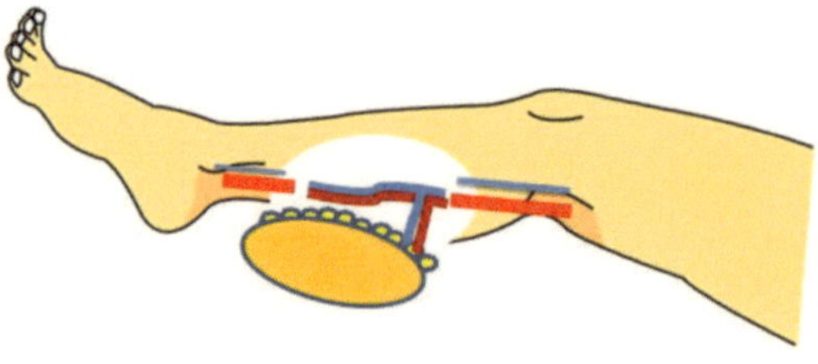

Figure 18. Schematic representation of the flow-through free flap procedure of vascular repair for Gustilo-Anderson IIIC fracture. This method makes both vascular repair and immediate wound resurfacing possible.

5. Discussion and conclusion

It is widely known that artificial dermis is used for the reconstruction of wounds with exposed tendons or bone, because it promotes early infiltration of mononuclear cells and fibroblasts and better growth of connective tissue strands and epithelium [10]. However, bone-exposing wounds in our patients with Gustilo-Anderson IIIB and C fractures had not improved with this treatment, and required conventional flap surgery. The main problem might have been the total absence or extreme deficiency of blood flow to bone fragment or fractured stumps, which had led to sequestration and osteomyelitis, prolonging the period of external fixation. Although the wounds might not have developed infection, a favorable wound bed could not have developed with poor vascularity. We conclude that, at the present stage of its development, artificial dermis is not a recommendable resurfacing option for patients with Gustilo-Anderson IIIB and C fractures, because it does not help improve poor bone circulation, a fact which may result in osteomyelitis. Thus, immediate primary skin closure is desired for patients with Gustilo-Anderson IIIB and C fractures [15].

6. Application of free flow-through anterolateral thigh (ATL) flap for Gustilo-Anderson IIIB and C bone-exposing wounds

6.1. Advantage of flow-through type flaps

The vascular injury associated with extremity trauma primarily requires open vascular repair immediate after injury, such as direct anastomosis, an interposition vein graft, or a bypass graft, to restore blood flow to distal area of injured extremities [13] (**Figure 17**). Since the development of concept of the flow-through flap, in which both the proximal and distal ends of the vascular pedicle of a free flap are anastomosed to restore blood flow to distal tissues, many investigators have described the application of flow-through flaps for reconstruction of the extremities [16–19] (**Figure 18**). Instead of conventional interposing vein graft to replace the injured artery, microsurgical free flow-through type flaps use has the added benefit of restoring blood flow to the distal extremities normally, whilst simultaneously immediately reconstructing soft-tissue defects in soft-tissue-deficient wounds. Furthermore, exploring the recipient vasculature for purpose of anastomosing the flap vessels is usually straightforward when reconstructive surgery is performed immediately after injury [20].

These special flaps require a T-shaped branching system of the pedicle vessel with proper diameters. Surgeon can choose several kinds of flow-through type flaps, including latissimus dorsi musculocutaneous, rectus abdominis musculocutaneous, fibula osteomyocutaneous, and anterolateral thigh (ALT) flaps [20–22]. Among all of the above, the ALT flap can provide a large skin paddle and long and suitable pedicle; thus, it is ideal for extremity reconstruction with minimal donor site morbidity [23]. In this article, we present cases of successful salvage and reconstruction of the extremities using free flow-through ALT flaps.

6.2. Case presentations of Gustilo-Anderson IIIB and C limb fractures reconstructed with free ALT flow-through type flaps

Case 7. Having been caught in a harvester, a 62-year-old man sustained a Gustilo-Anderson type IIIC ulnar fracture to the left elbow with wide abrasion of the skin and flexor muscles (**Figure 19**) defect in the ulna, with subsequent opening of the elbow joint cavity (**Figure 20**). The circulation of the left forearm had ceased due to interruption of the brachial artery (**Figure 21**). Immediate reconstruction using a free ALT flow-through type flap was performed. After debridement and external fixation of the elbow joint, the T portion of the descending branch of the lateral circumflex femoral

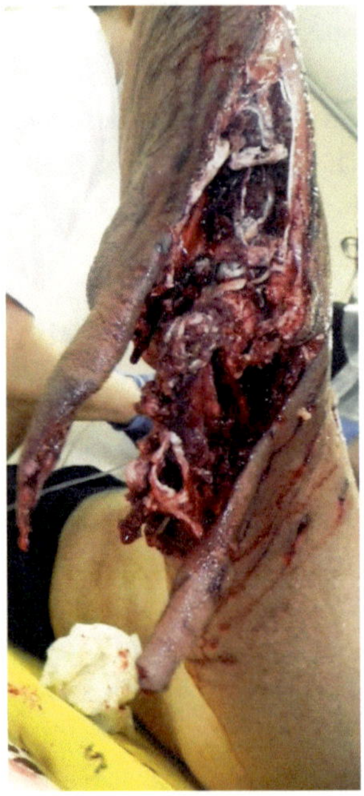

Figure 19. Case 5. The picture shows Gustilo-Anderson IIIC fracture to the left elbow with abrasion of the skin and flexor muscles.

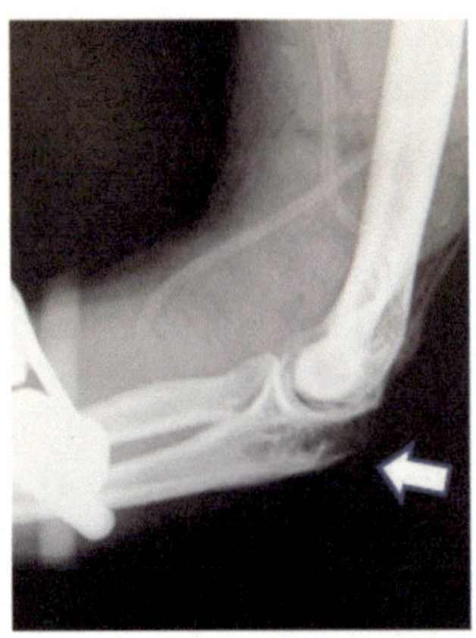

Figure 20. An X-ray photograph shows bone defect of ulna, which caused opening of elbow joint cavity.

http://dx.doi.org/10.5772/intechopen.70147

artery was interposed within the defect of the brachial artery. Two veins were connected to the cutaneous veins by end-to-end anastomosis (**Figures 22** and **23**). The defect of elbow joint capsule was reconstructed with the fascia of the ALT flap, and the bone- and joint-exposing wound was

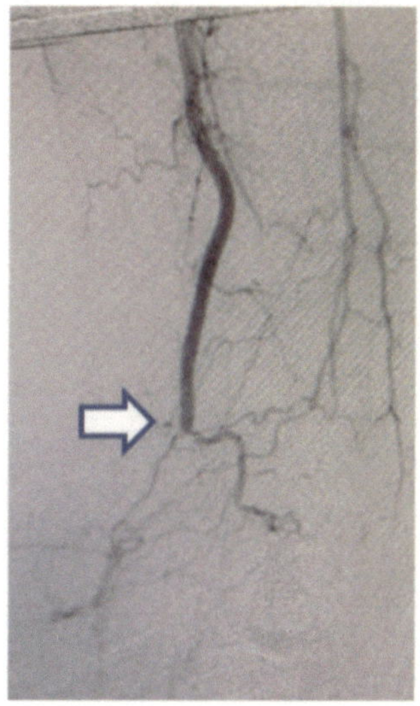

Figure 21. Contrast-enhanced computed tomography showed that circulation of the left forearm had ceased due to interruption of brachial artery.

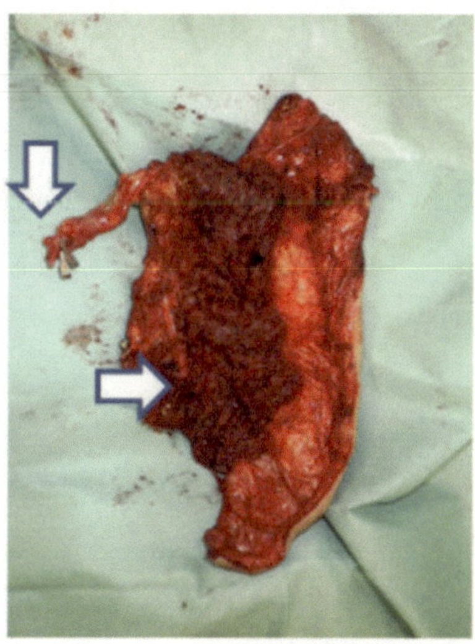

Figure 22. The picture shows a harvested flow-through ALT flap. Arrows indicate the distal and proximal ends of the descending branch.

resurfaced with the vastus lateralis overlying skin island. The blood flow to the hand and forearm through the interposed descending branch was restored, while that to the flap was also favorable (**Figure 24**). The patient could flex his elbow 3 months after surgery (**Figures 25**).

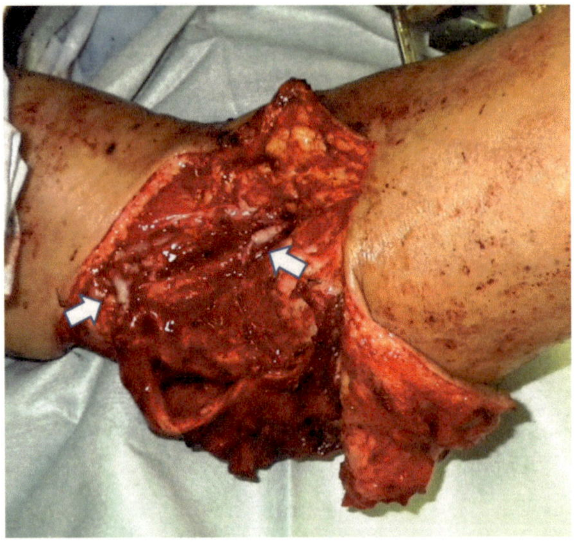

Figure 23. The intraoperative photograph shows the descending branch interposed within the interrupted brachial artery. Arrows indicate the areas of anastomosis.

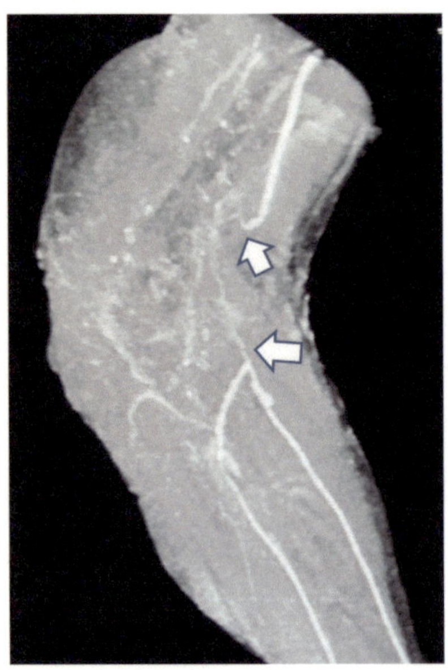

Figure 24. Contrast-enhanced computed tomography 2 weeks after surgery showing reestablishment of circulation to the hand and forearm through the interposed descending branch, and blood flow to the flap. The arrows indicated the points of anastomosis.

http://dx.doi.org/10.5772/intechopen.70147

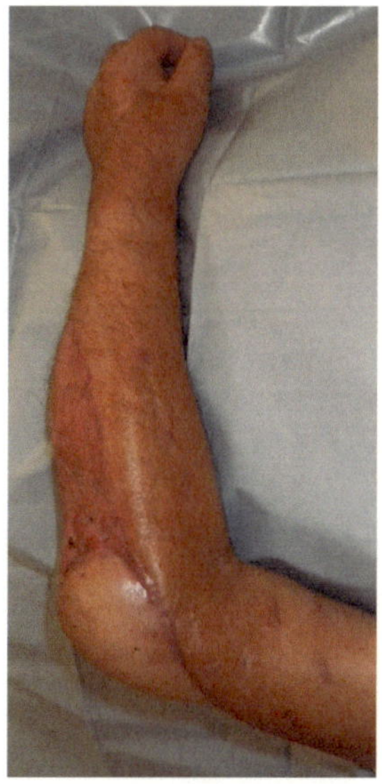

Figure 25. View of the reconstructed forearm 3 month after surgery showing favorable resurfacing and successful functional outcome.

Case 8: Due to a traffic accident, a 32-year-old man sustained a Gustilo-Anderson IIIC type bone-exposing fracture to the left fibula and tibia with severe abrasion of the skin and anterior tibial muscles (**Figure 26**). Circulation of the left foot had ceased because three main arteries

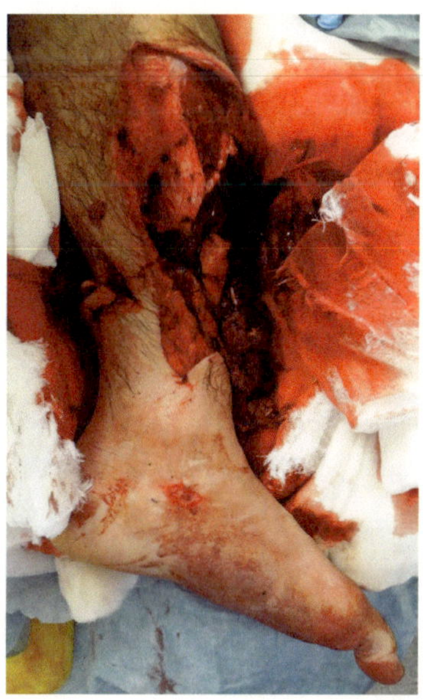

Figure 26. Case 6. This photograph shows a Gustilo-Anderson IIIC fracture to the left fibula and tibia with severe abrasion of the skin and anterior tibial muscles.

in the leg (peroneal, posterior tibial, and anterior tibial arteries) had ruptured, and flow had been interrupted. After the crushed bones had been reconstructed and fixed externally, the bone-exposing wound was repaired with a free flow-through ALT flap (**Figures 27** and **28**). The T portion of the descending branch of the ALT flap was interposed to the defect of the anterior tibia artery, and two veins were connected to the cutaneous veins by end-to-end anastomosis. The interrupted anterior tibia artery resumed normal blood flow (**Figure 29**). The viability of the flap was favorable without infection and necrosis. The patient could walk without canes 1 year after surgery (**Figures 30** and **31**).

6.3. Discussion and conclusion

A flow-through flap is utilized when the flap inflow arterial system not only provides perfusion to the transported flap but also provides a vascular link between the obliterated arteries [24, 25]. Especially, this flap is useful for patients suffering from Gustilo-Anderson IIIC complex injuries, which present with both large soft-tissue defects and main artery defects with compromised circulation of a distal extremities. The flow-through flap transfer can be superior to conventional flaps for achieving the resurfacing of a large tissue defect and vascular repair immediately, a process which reduces infection, induces bony healing, and optimizes limb salvage [23].

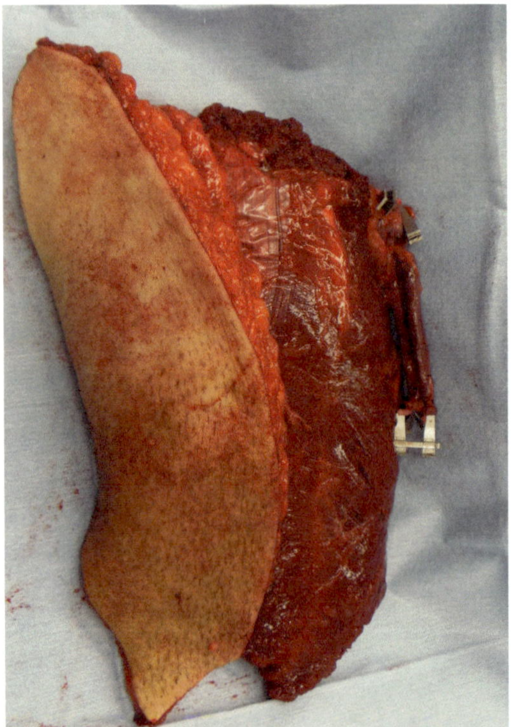

Figure 27. This picture shows a harvested flow-through ALT flap.

http://dx.doi.org/10.5772/intechopen.70147

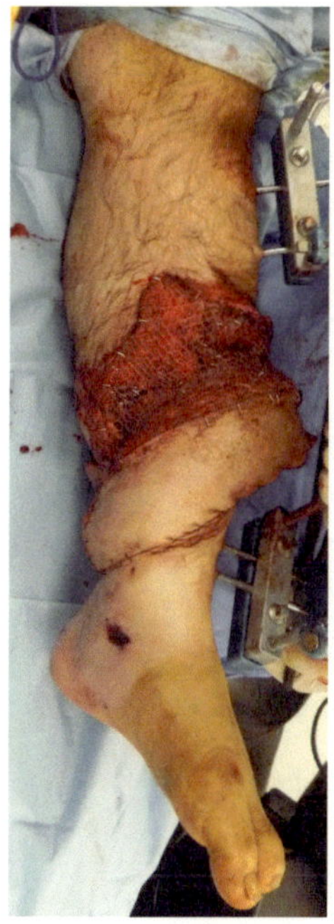

Figure 28. A The postoperative photograph showing resurfacing with flap and skin graft; circulation of the foot resumed immediately.

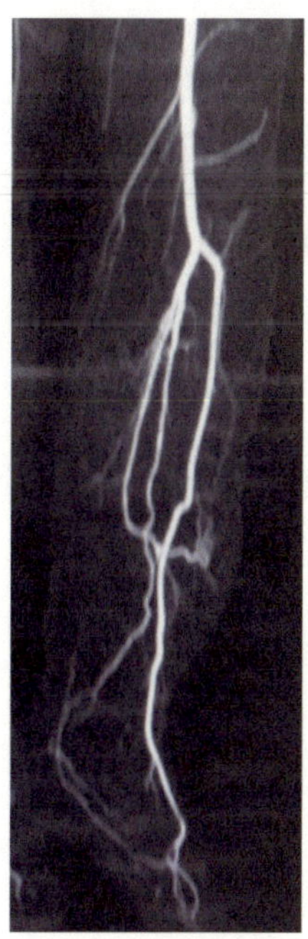

Figure 29. Computed tomography angiography reveals that the descending branch of the ALT flap was interposed into the defect of the anterior tibia artery, which supplied blood flow to the foot.

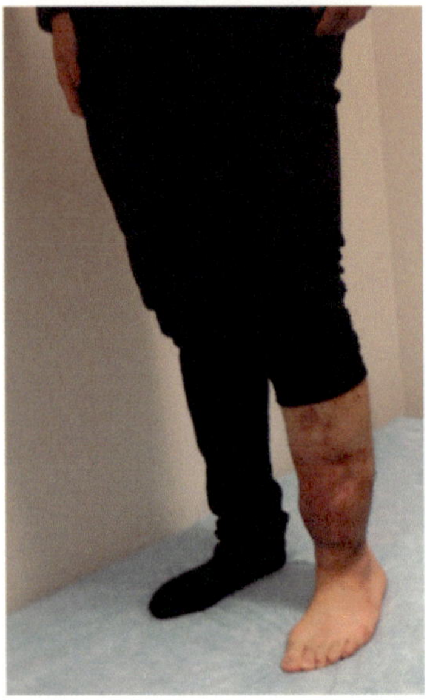

Figure 30. The patient could walk without canes1 year after surgery.

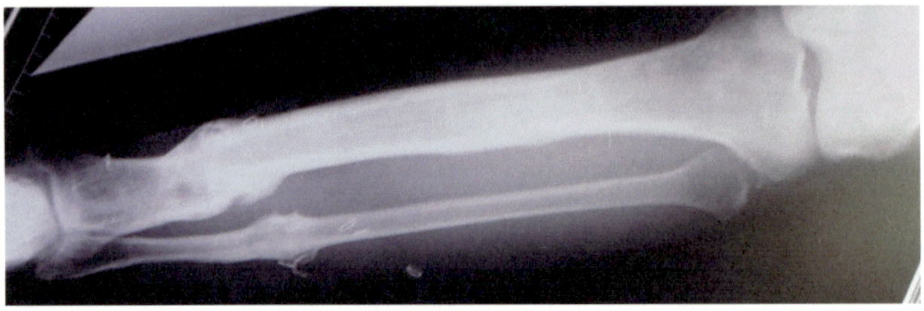

Figure 31. An X-ray photograph shows favorable bone union.

7. "Fix and flap," a new radical concept for the treatment of severe open fractures

7.1. Concept of "fix and flap" procedure for open fracture

Wound closure of severe open fractures has been delayed with the aim to minimize the risk of infection. However, development of systemic antibiotics, advanced debridement methods, and improvement of surgical techniques have reduced surgical infection. As recent studies have reported that infections after treatment of open fractures are not caused by initial contamination but often are acquired later, emergent or early wound resurfacing for open fractures has been recommended [26–29]. On the other hand, a new radical concept for the treatment of severe open fractures so-called "fix and flap" is recommended as this method also reduces infection [30–32].

http://dx.doi.org/10.5772/intechopen.70147

7.2. Case presentation of fix and flap procedure for Gustilo-Anderson IIIB fracture

A 32-year-old man sustained Gustilo-Anderson IIIB type both tibia and fibula fractures to the right leg with abrasion of the skin and hamstring muscles (**Figures 32** and **33**). After immediate cleansing, reduction, and temporary external fixation, the secondary "fix and

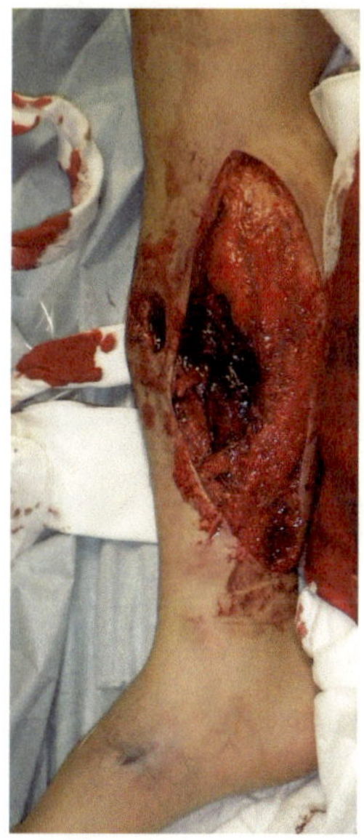

Figure 32. Case 7. This photograph shows a Gustilo-Anderson IIIB type bone-exposing fracture to the right leg with abrasion of the skin and hamstring muscles.

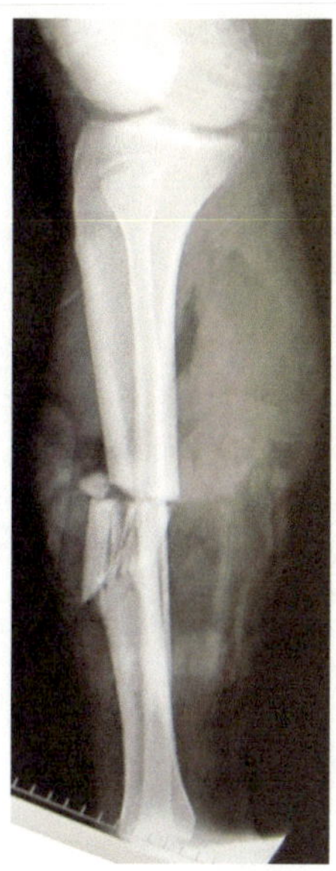

Figure 33. An X-ray photograph shows both tibia and fibula fractures.

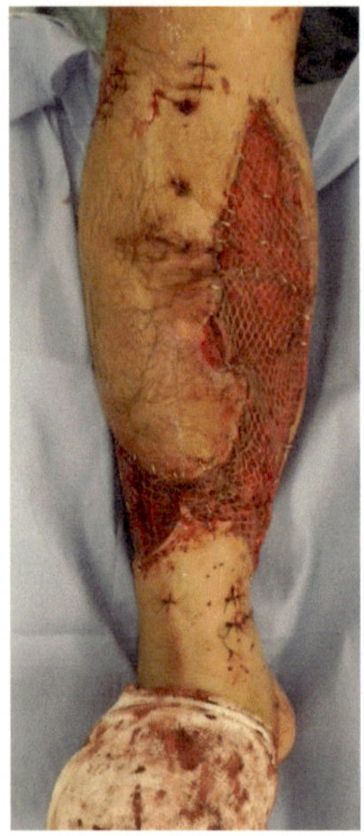

Figure 34. Late "fix and flap" surgery including internal bone fixation, local frap transfer; a free skin graft was performed 5 days later.

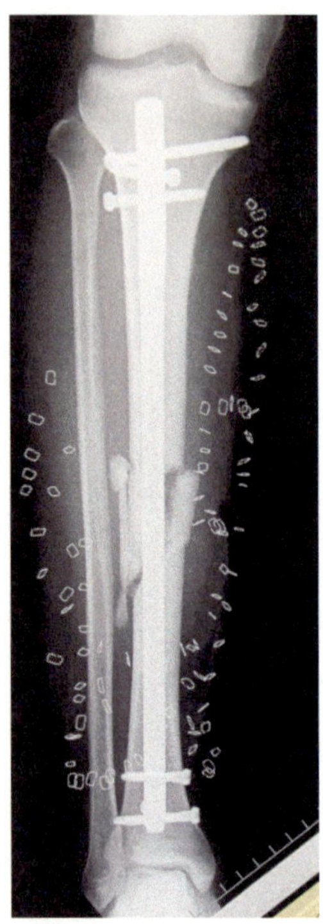

Figure 35. An X-ray photograph showing ridged fixation of the broken tibia using intramedullary fixation system.

flap" surgery including internal bone fixation, fasciocutaneous frap transfer, and free skin graft was performed 5 days later (**Figure 34**). The wound was healed 10 days later, the patient could walk 1 month after secondary surgery without cane because rigid intramedullary fixation system conferred steady stability to the broken leg (**Figures 35** and **36**).

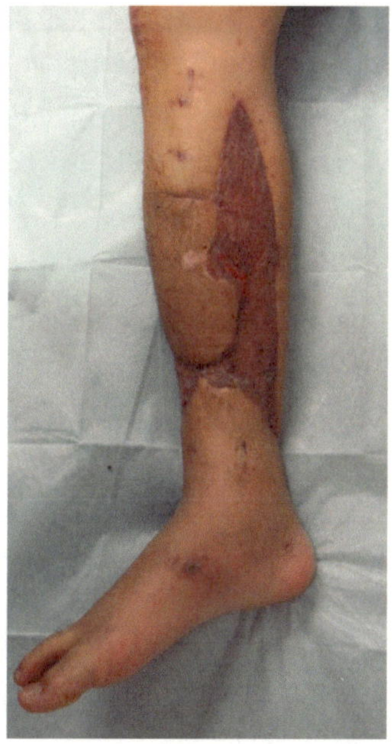

Figure 36. View of the reconstructed leg 1 month after surgery, showing favorable resurfacing.

8. Conclusion

Surgeons are recommended to perform early closure of the wound after rigid bone fixation. These "fix and flap" procedures improve postsurgical problems such as infection, and accelerate the rehabilitation, a process which speeds up patients' recovery and improve their quality of life [30–32].

Author details

Masaki Fujioka

Address all correspondence to: mfujioka@nagasaki-mc.com

Department of Plastic and Reconstructive Surgery, Clinical Research Center, National Hospital Organization Nagasaki Medical Center, Nagasaki, Japan

References

[1] Gustilo RB, Anderson JT. Prevention of infection in the treatment of one thousand and twenty-five open fractures of long bones: Retrospective and prospective analyses. The Journal of Bone and Joint Surgery American. 1976;**58**:453-458

[2] Clancey GJ, Hansen Jr ST. Open fractures of the tibia: A review of one hundred and two cases. The Journal of Bone and Joint Surgery American. 1978;**60-A**:118-122

[3] Russell GG, Henderson R, Arnett G. Primary or delayed closure for open tibial fractures. Journal of Bone and Joint Surgery, British. 1990;**72-B**:125-128

[4] Goldner JL, Hardaker Jr WT, Mabrey JD. Open fractures of the extremities: The case for open treatment. Postgraduate Medical. 1985;**78**:199-214

[5] Trueta J. Reflections on the past and present treatment of war wounds and fractures. Military Medicine. 1976;**141**:255-258

[6] Chen X, Chen H, Zhang G. Management of wounds with exposed bone structures using an artificial dermis and skin grafting technique. Journal of Plastic, Reconstructive & Aesthetic Surgery. 2010;**63**(6):e512-518

[7] Fujioka M. Artificial dermis: A new material for wound treatment. Journal of Wound Technology. 2009;**4**:13-19

[8] Fujioka M. Combination treatment with basic fibroblast growth factor and artificial dermis improves complex wounds caused by collagen diseases with steroid use. Dermatologic Surgery. 2009;**35**(9):1422-1425

[9] Daniel RS, Adam GH, Lawrence XW. Negative pressure wound therapy in grade IIIB tibial fractures: Fewer infections and fewer flap procedures? Clinical Orthopaedics and Related Research. 2015;**473**(5):1802-1811. DOI: 10.1007/s11999-015-4140-1

[10] Hom DB, Manivel JC. Promoting healing with recombinant human platelet-derived growth factor–BB in a previously irradiated problem wound. Laryngoscope. 2003;**113**: 1566-1571

[11] Fujioka M, Fujii T. Maxillary growth following atelocollagen implantation on mucoperiosteal denudation of the palatal process in young rabbits: Implications for clinical cleft palate repair. The Cleft Palate-Craniofacial Journal. 1997;**34**:297-308

[12] Soni A, Tzafetta K, Knight S, Giannoudis PV. Gustilo IIIC fractures in the lower limb: Our 15-year experience. Journal of Bone and Joint Surgery, British. 2012;**94**:698-703

[13] Halvorson JJ, Anz A, Langfitt M, Deonanan JK, Scott A, Teasdall RD, Carroll EA, Carroll EA. Vascular injury associated with extremity trauma: Initial diagnosis and management. Journal of the American Academy of Orthopaedic Surgeons. 2011;**19**:495-504

[14] Fujioka M, Hayashida K, Murakami C. Artificial dermis is not effective for resurfacing the bone-exposing wounds of Gustilo-Anderson III fracture. Journal of Plastic, Reconstructive & Aesthetic Surgery. 2013;**66**:e119-e121

[15] Rajasekaran S, Dheenadhayalan J, Babu JN, Sundararajan SR, Venkatramani H, Sabapathy SR. Immediate primary skin closure in type-III A and B open fractures: Results after a minimum of five years. Journal of Bone and Joint Surgery, British. 2009;**91**(2):217-224. DOI: 10.1302/0301-620X.91B2.21228

[16] Soutar DS, Scheker LR, Tanner NS, McGregor IA. The radial forearm flap: A versatile method for intra-oral reconstruction. British Journal of Plastic Surgery. 1983;**36**(1):1-8

[17] Koshima I, Fujitsu M, Ushio S, Sugiyama N, Yamashita S. Flow-through anterior thigh flaps with a short pedicle for reconstruction of lower leg and foot defects. Plastic and Reconstructive Surgery. 2005;**115**(1):155162

[18] Miyamoto S, Kayano S, Umezawa H, Fujiki M, Sakuraba M. Flow-through fibula flap using soleus branch as distal runoff: A case report. Microsurgery. 2013;**33**(1):60-62

[19] Garvey PB, Clemens MW, Rhines LD, Sacks JM. Vertical rectus abdominis musculo-cutaneous flow-through flap to a free fibula flap for total sacrectomy reconstruction. Microsurgery. 2013;**33**(1):32-38

[20] Kim JT, Kim CY, Kim YH. T-anastomosis in microsurgical free flap reconstruction: an overview of clinical applications. Journal of Plastic, Reconstructive & Aesthetic Surgery. 2008;**61**(10):1157-1163

[21] Rowsell AR, Davies DM, Eisenberg N, Taylor GI. The anatomy of the subscapular-thoracodorsal arterial system: study of 100 cadaver dissections. British Journal of Plastic Surgery. 1984;**37**(4):574-576

[22] Xu DC, Zhong SZ, Kong JM, et al. Applied anatomy of the anterolateral femoral flap. Plastic and Reconstructive Surgery. 1988;**82**(2):305-310

[23] Fujioka M, Hayashida K, Murakami C. Emergent free flow-through anterolateral thigh flaps for Gustilo-Anderson III fracture of the upper extremity. Journal of Emergencies, Trauma and Shock. 2014;**7**(1):53-55. DOI: 10.4103/0974-2700.125642

[24] Hidalgo DA. Aesthetic improvements in free-flap mandible reconstruction. Plastic and Reconstructive Surgery. 1991;**88**:574-585

[25] Saint-Cyr M, Langstein HN. Reconstruction of the hand and upper extremity after tumor resection. Journal of Surgical Oncology. 2006;**94**:490-503

[26] Weitz-Marshall AD, Bosse MJ. Timing of closure of open fractures. Journal of the American Academy of Orthopaedic Surgeons. 2002;**10**:379-384

[27] Moola F, Jacks D, Reindl R, Berry G, Harvey EJ. Safety of primary closure of soft tissue wounds in open fractures. Journal of Bone and Joint Surgery, British. 2008;**90-B**(Suppl 1):94

[28] Hohmann E, Tetsworth K, Radziejowski MJ, Wiesniewski TF. Comparison of delayed and primary wound closure in the treatment of open tibial fractures. Archives of Orthopaedic and Trauma Surgery. 2007;**127**:131-136

[29] Siwach R, Singh R, Arya S, Gupta R. Treatment of 78 type II and type IIIa open fractures by primary closure on suction drain: A prospective study. Journal of Orthopaedic Trauma. 2007;**8**:173-176

[30] DeLong Jr WG, Born CT, Wei SY, et al. Aggressive treatment of 119 open fracture wounds. The Journal of Trauma 1999;**46**:1049-1054.

[31] Gopal S, Majumder S, Batchelor AG, et al. Fix and flap: The radical orthopaedic and plastic treatment of severe open fractures of the tibia. Journal of Bone and Joint Surgery, British. 2000;**82-B**:959-966

[32] Hertel R, Lambert SM, Muller S, Ballmer FT, Ganz R. On the timing of soft tissue reconstruction for open fractures of the lower leg. Archives of Orthopaedic and Trauma Surgery. 1999;**119**:7-12

Section 3

Special Situations

Chapter 6

Reconstruction for Mandibular Implant Failure

Shih-Heng Chen, Hao-Chih Tai, Tai-Ju Cheng,
Hung-Chi Chen, An-Ta Ko, Tyng-Luan Roan,
Yo-Shen Chen and Yueh-Bih Tang

Additional information is available at the end of the chapter

http://dx.doi.org/10.5772/intechopen.70166

Abstract

Mandibular defects may result from tumor ablations, trauma, or radiation necrosis. Significant segmental mandibular loss or hemimandibular loss may sometimes be replaced with mandibular implants by ENT surgeons/oral surgeons/head and neck surgeons. However, this may bring about mandibular implant failure in long-term follow-up. Mandibular implant failures usually manifest as: soft tissue atrophy, mandibular implant extrusion, infection, facial nerve involvement, facial asymmetry, derangement of occlusion and mastication, orocutaneous fistula, etc. Over 30 years, the authors have treated 102 patients with mandibular implant failure. Reconstruction may involve removal of the mandibular implant and immediate replacement of the mandibular defect with a piece of vascularized bone flap, not only to compensate for bone loss but also to replace neighboring soft tissue and possible skin defects. Frequently used flaps have been vascularized iliac bone (89/102) or vascularized fibula grafts (13/102). During follow-up, iliac bone flap reconstruction has yielded more favorable results due to its ample bone bulk and adequate soft tissue coverage. Fibula flaps with osteotomies have been associated with an increasing incidence of malunion/nonunion and subsequent easy deformation.

Keywords: mandibular reconstruction, implant failures, vascularized iliac bone flap, vascularized fibula bone flap, finesse

1. Introduction

Mandibular defects may result from tumor ablations, trauma, or radiation necrosis. Significant segmental mandibular loss or hemimandibular loss may be replaced with mandibular implants by head and neck surgeons or oral surgeons in order to terminate surgery quickly [1]. However, mandibular implant failure may ensue on long-term follow-up.

The cause of mandibular implant failure may be related to high functional demands on mastication, speech, yawning, and singing. The force and pressures imposed on the mandible by chewing, yawning, and mouth opening make mandibular implants liable to extrusion sooner or later.

Complications of mandibular implant include infection, loosening, deformation, soft tissue wasting, extrusion, capsular contracture, and sometimes the development of a skin defect owing to infection with subsequent scar contracture (**Table 1**).

Infection
Extrusion
Malocclusion
Soft tissue wasting
Loosening of implant
Facial nerve involvement
Deformation of lower face

Table 1. Mandibular implant failures.

2. Manifestations

1. Facial deformities
   a. Soft tissue wasting (**Figure 1**)
   b. Deformation (**Figures 2** and **3**)
   c. Deviation of mandible and chin (**Figure 4**)
2. Extrusion of mandibular implant (**Figure 5**)
3. Infection (**Figure 6**)
4. Orocutaneous fistula (**Figure 7(a)**: extrusion of mandibular implant intraorally, (7b): mandibular implant at symphysis, **Figure 7(c)**: orocutaneous fistula)

http://dx.doi.org/10.5772/intechopen.70166

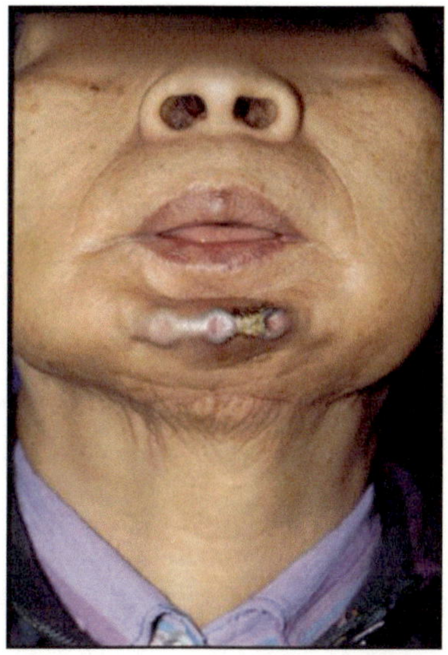

Figure 1. Soft tissue wasting.

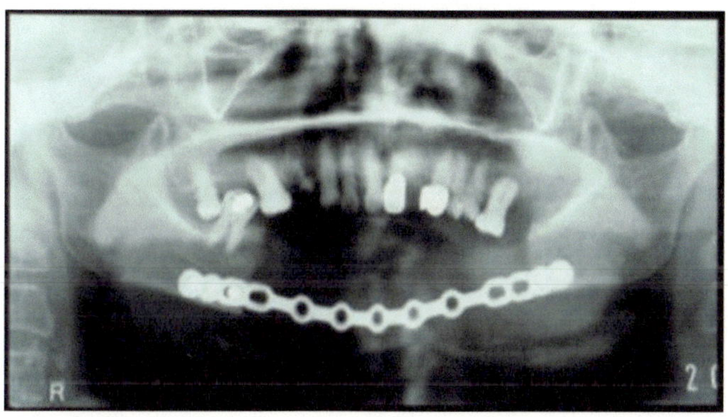

Figure 2. Immediate after operation.

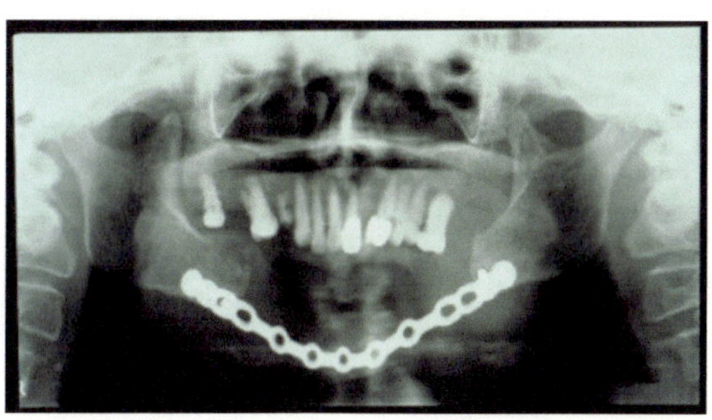

Figure 3. Angulation deformity 1 year after operation.

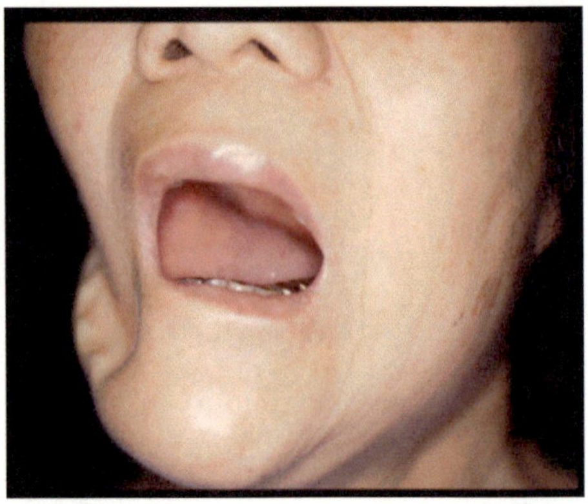

Figure 4. Deviation of mandible and chin.

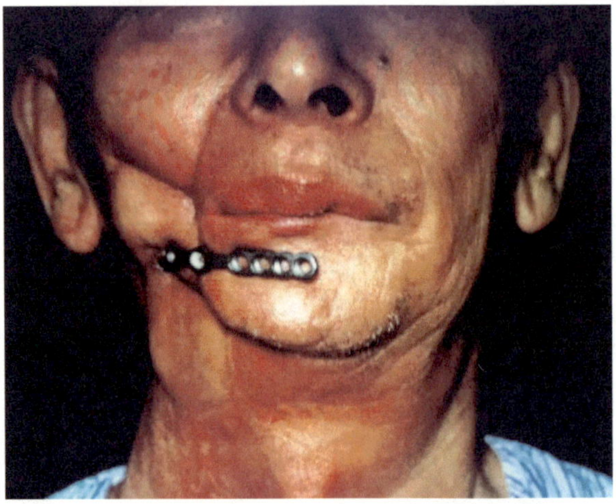

Figure 5. Extrusion of mandibular implant.

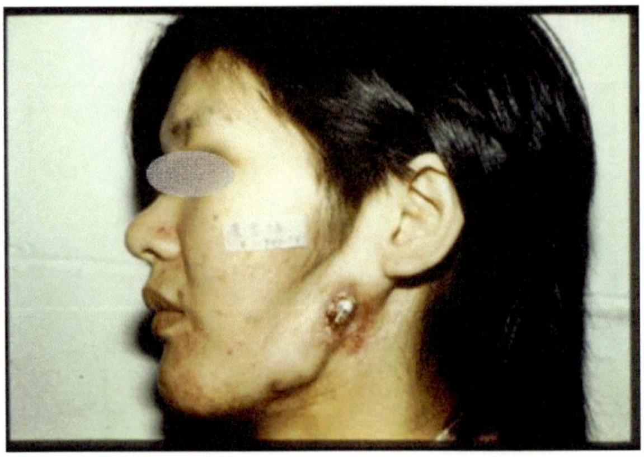

Figure 6. Mandibular implant extrusion with infection.

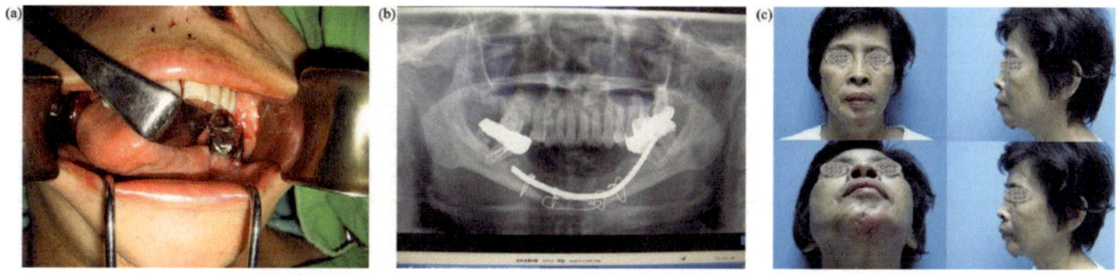

Figure 7. (a) Extrusion of mandibular implant intraorally. (b) Mandibular implant at symphysis. (c) Orocutaneous fistula.

3. Patients and methods

During the past 35 years, 102 patients with mandibular implant failures had been referred for further treatments (**Table 2**) [2].

The manifestations were

1. Facial deformities

   Significant facial deformities usually brought the patients to seek plastic surgeons.

   a. Soft tissue wasting (**Figure 8**)

   b. Deviation of mandible and chin (**Figure 9**)

2. Extrusion of mandibular implant

   Extrusion occurred intraorally (**Figure 10(a)**) or extraorally (**Figure 10(b)**)

3. Infection

   Infection ensued with or without extrusion of mandibular implant (**Figure 11(a)** and **(b)**)

4. Orocutaneous fistula (**Figure 12**)

   Orocutaneous fistula occurred when intraoral extrusion of the implant brought saliva passing by the implant, causing infection. This was soon supervened with an orocutaneous fistula, which never healed.

Removal of implant	36
Total	32
Partial	4
Retention of implant	66
Reconstruction with	
Vascularized iliac bone	83
Vascularized fibula	19

Table 2. Method.

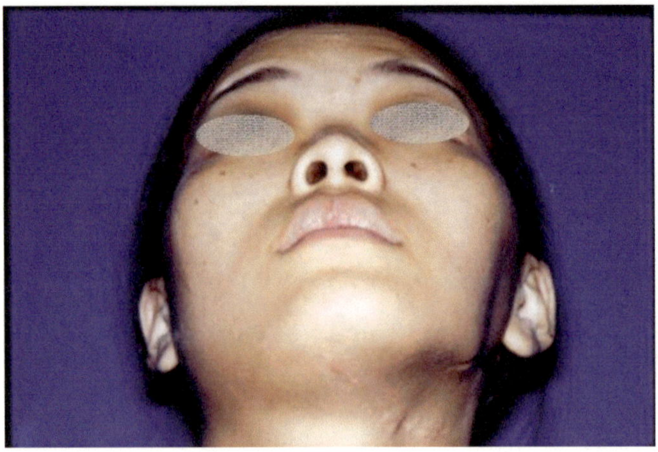

Figure 8. Soft tissue wasting at left side lower face.

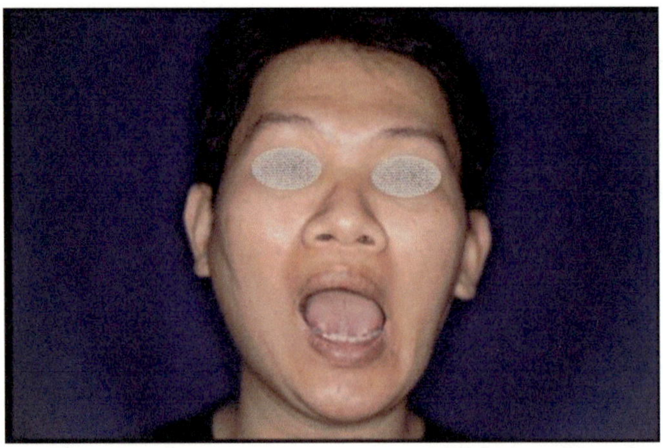

Figure 9. Deviation of mandible and chin.

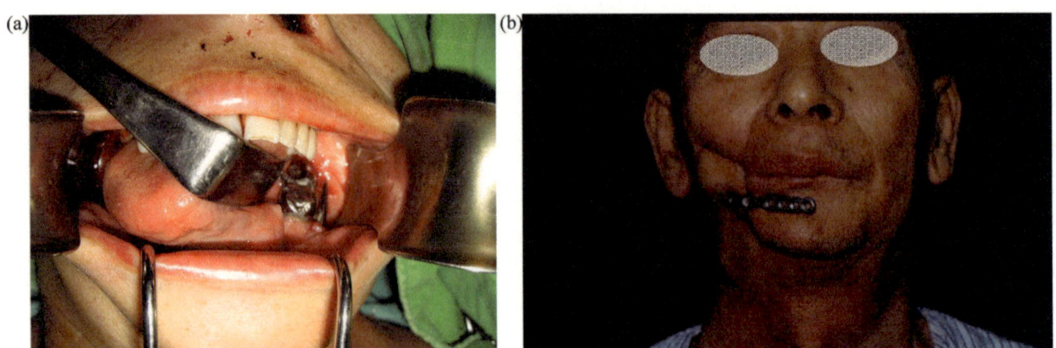

Figure 10. (a) Extrusion of mandibular implant intraorally. (b) Extrusion of mandibular implant extraorally.

http://dx.doi.org/10.5772/intechopen.70166

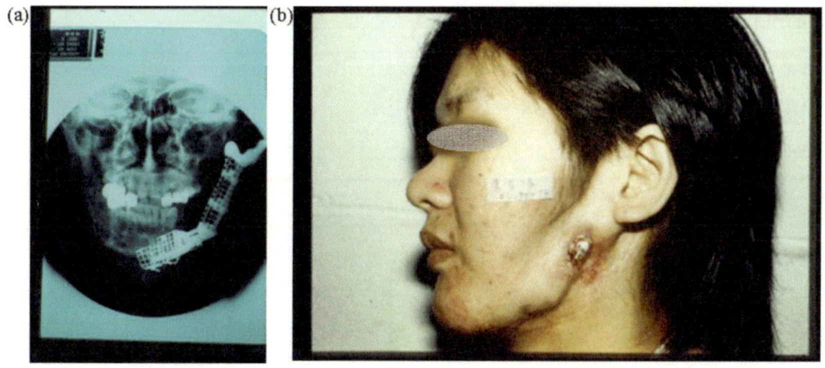

Figure 11. (a) Left mandibular implant. (b) Extrusion of mandibular implant with infection.

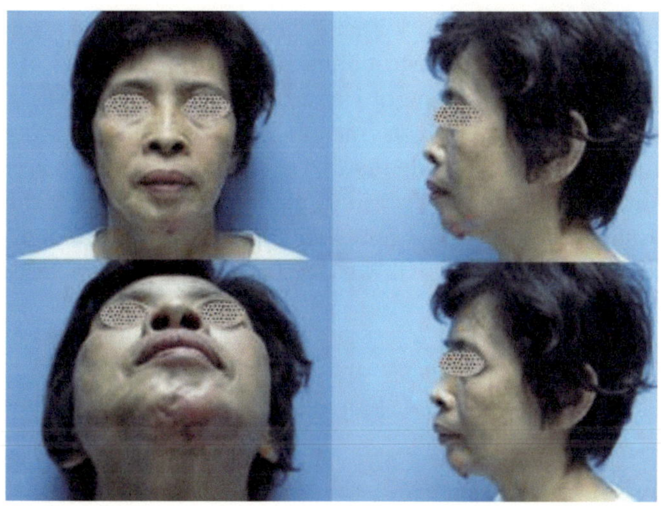

Figure 12. Orocutaneous fistula.

4. Strategy of treatment

I. Removal of mandibular implant when the implant became extruded or got infected [3].

II. Immediate reconstruction of missing mandibular segment or hemimandible with vascularized bone, incorporating soft tissue and skin flap for intraoral mucosal lining/external skin defect reconstruction/replacement of soft tissue defect. The vascularized bone can be an iliac bone flap or fibula flap [4, 5]. Selection of vascularized bone (**Table 3**)

   A. Hemimandibular defect: vascularized iliac bone [2, 6–8].

   With implant retained *in situ* in patients without implant extrusion.

   With implant removed in patients with implant extrusion.

B. Segmental defect

Iliac bone flap was more preferable than fibular flap due to more bony height with ample soft tissue and skin paddle [7–10].

C. Anterior mandibular defect: vascularized iliac bone

D. Lateral segment defect: fibula flap [5]

III. Repositioning of skin flap

Banked external skin flap could be moved intraorally after the subsidence of tissue swelling.

IV. Reshaping of bony contour

After bony union, some imperfect bony contour may be reshaped [4].

V. Removal of the mandibular plate

VI. For nearly hemimandibular reconstructions, overzealous removal of the reconstruction plate for further reconstruction might jeopardize the overlying facial nerve which had already been surrounded by fibrosis and might have assumed a nonanatomical path. Thereafter, surgical manipulation in this area to create space might stretch the facial nerve overlying the implant and might lead to its inadvertent injury. For this reason, the plate was either partially removed or not removed at all as long as it had not been already become extruded or infected; instead, it was overlaid with a piece of vascularized bone flap.

I. Removal of Mandibular implant when the implant become or got in fected.
II. Immediate reconstruction of missing mandibular segment.
(A) Hemimandibular defect:
Vascularized iliac bone
With implant retained *in situ*
With implant removed (total or partial)
(B) Segmental defect:
Iliac bone flap is more preferable than fibular flap due to more bony height
(C) Anterior mandibular defect:
Vascularized iliac bone
(D) Lateral segment defect:
Fibula flap
III. Reposition of skin flap
Banked external skin flap can be moved inwardly with subsidence of tissue swelling
IV. Reshaping of bony contour
After bony union, some imperfect bony contour may be reshaped

Table 3. Summary of operation technique.

5. Problems of reconstruction with implant failure and removal of the implant

1. Scarring and capsule formation around the implant.
2. Difficulty in dissecting and approaching the glenoid fossa.
3. Lack of a clear plane to expand the pocket to accommodate a vascularized bone mimicking the ascending ramus.
4. Possibility of facial nerve injury or traction during dissection or expansion.
5. Placement of incision should be carefully designed since there had been soft tissue atrophy and thinning of skin (**Figure 13(a)** and **(b)**).

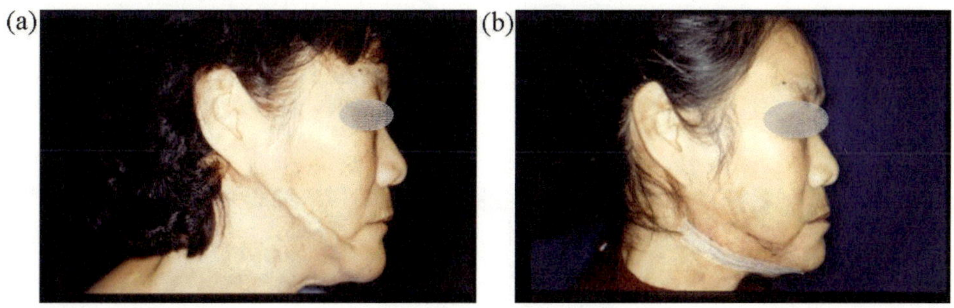

Figure 13. (a) Thinning of skin overlying mandibular implant. (b) Reconstruction with iliac bone flap with upper neck transverse incision.

6. Case presentations

A. Hemimandibular reconstruction with mandibular tray implant (**Figure 14(a–d)**).

1. Removal of mandibular implant.
2. Immediate hemimandibular reconstruction with vascularized iliac bone flap.
3. Fascia lata sling operation to hold the mandibular body to temporal muscle and fascia.
4. Facial recontouring, soft tissue, and bone.

B. Facial asymmetry after resection of mandibular ameloblastoma and mere reconstruction with mandibular reconstruction plate (**Figure 15(a)** and **(b)**).

C. Young man, aged 25 years, suffered from soft tissue wasting 1 year after sole mandibular implant insertion and his status after subcondylar mandibular reconstruction (**Figure 16(a–d)**).

D. Young man, aged 28 years, suffered from soft tissue wasting and chin deviation 6 months after resection of a left side mandibular ameloblastoma and subsequent reconstruction with

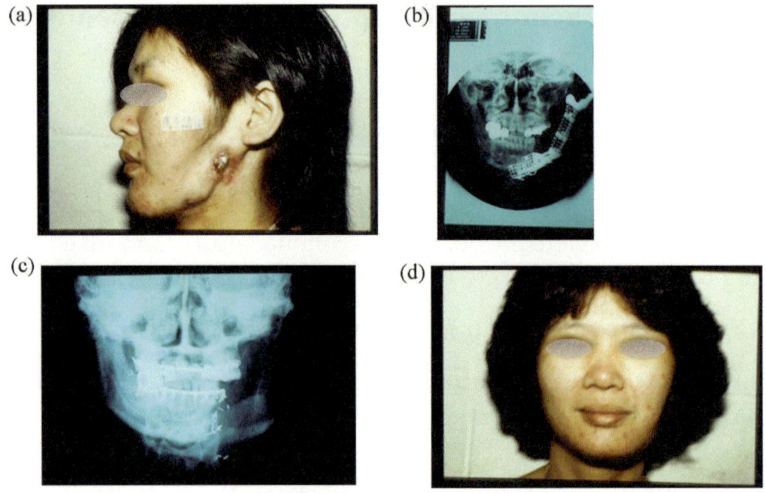

Figure 14. (a) Extrusion of mandibular implant with infection, soft tissue wasting and facial deformity. (b) Preoperative roentgenography. (c) Postoperative roentgenography after reconstruction with vascularized iliac bone flap. (d) Postoperative photo showing satisfactory facial contour.

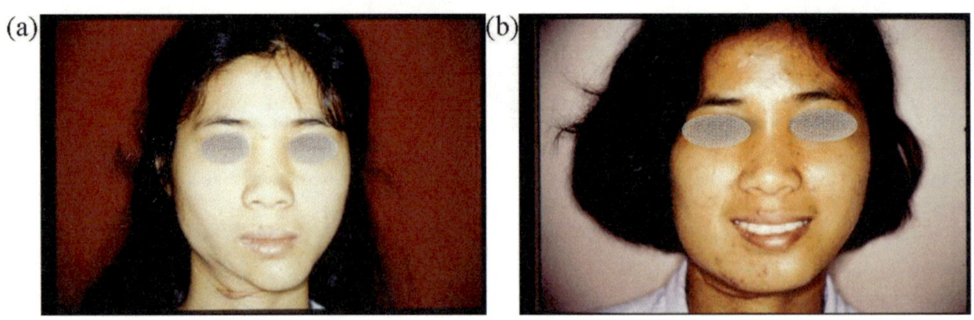

Figure 15. (a) Deformation of right side mandibular implant with deviation of chin. (b) Reconstruction with iliac bone flap, regained more symmetric facial contour.

mandibular reconstruction plate only (**Figure 17(a)**). He received mandibular reconstruction with retention of implant by onlaying a vascularized iliac bone flap on the reconstruction plate with osteosynthesis at the medial end of the mandibular section margin (**Figure 17(b)** and **(c)**). Picture 15 years after left hemimandibular reconstruction by an onlaying vascularized iliac bone flap on the reconstruction plate. No soft tissue atrophy or wasting was noticed. Occlusion was satisfactory with symmetric facial expression (**Figure 17(d)**).

E. This 24-year-old lady suffered from left side facial wasting after sub-hemimandibular reconstruction with reconstruction plate only (**Figure 18(a)**). She received mandibular reconstruction with an onlaying vascularized iliac bone flap with retaining the titanium reconstruction plate (**Figure 18**(**b–d**)).

F. A 66-year-old lady suffered from soft tissue wasting, deformation with impending extrusion of the implant 1 year after reconstructing a segmental symphyseal defect with a titanium mandibular reconstruction plate (**Figure 18(a–c)**). Removal of anterior segment mandibular implant and reconstruction with an iliac bone flap resulted in satisfactory bone union and facial contour (**Figure 18(d)**).

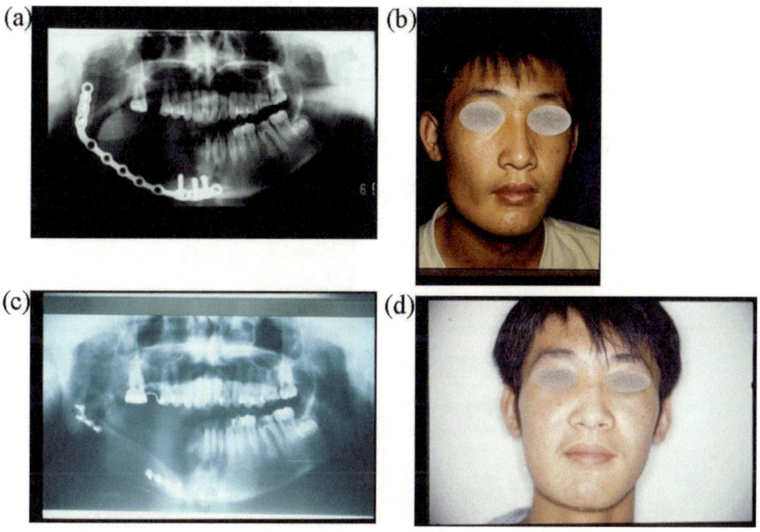

Figure 16. (a) Mandibular implant only, subcondylar hemimandibular reconstruction. (b) Soft tissue wasting 1 year after mandibular implant only subcondylar mandibular reconstruction. (c) Removal of reconstruction plate and replacement with vascularized iliac bone flap. (d) Postoperative photograph, s/p removal of reconstruction plate and replacement with vascularized iliac bone flap.

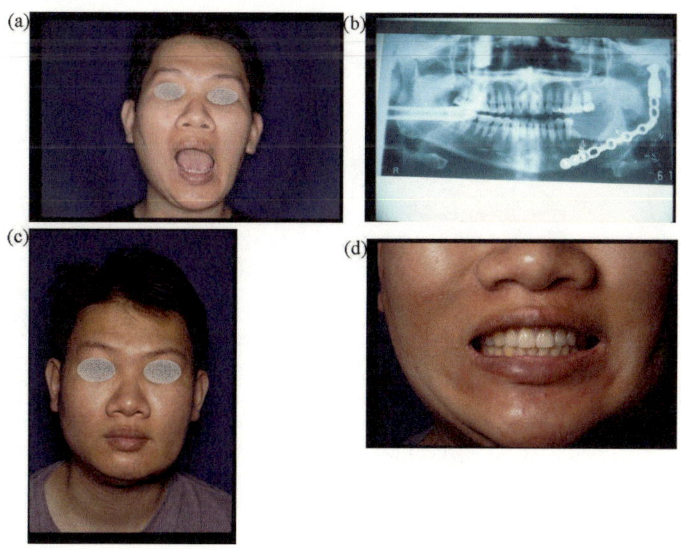

Figure 17. (a) Soft tissue wasting with deviation of chin. (b) Reconstruction was performed with retention of implant by onlaying a vascularized iliac bone flap on the reconstruction plate with osteosynthesis at the medial extreme. (c) Postoperative photography. (d) 15 years after left hemimandibular reconstruction by onlaying vascularized iliac bone flap on reconstruction plate, no soft tissue atrophy, wasting noticed. Occlusion was satisfactory with symmetric facial expression.

G. This 27-year-old young man received a hemimandibular implant reconstruction after resection of an ameloblastoma. However, it was complicated with infection and extrusion and ended up with implant removal, leaving a significant facial deformity (**Figure 19(a)**). The lateral segment mandibular defect was reconstructed with a fibula flap imcorporating with a titanium mandicular condyle (**Figure 19(b)** and **(c)**) [5].

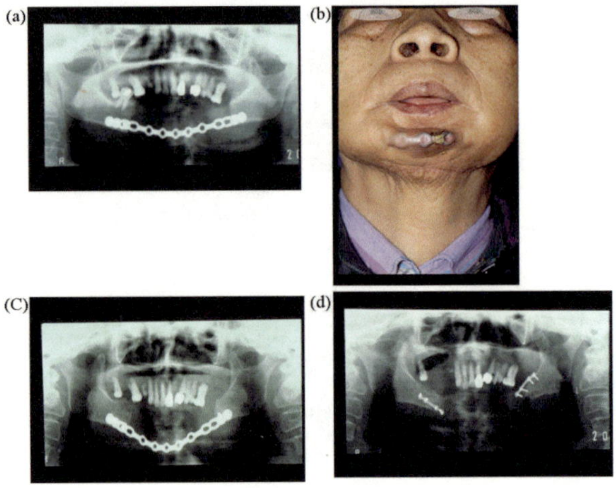

Figure 18. (a) Reconstruction plate only for reconstruction of symphyseal defect after resection of mandibular ameloblastoma. (b) Impending extrusion of symphyseal reconstruction plate. (c) Panex at 1 year post operation showing deformation of mandibular reconstruction plate. (d) Removal of anterior segment mandibular implant and reconstruction with iliac bone flap resulted in satisfactory bone union and facial contour.

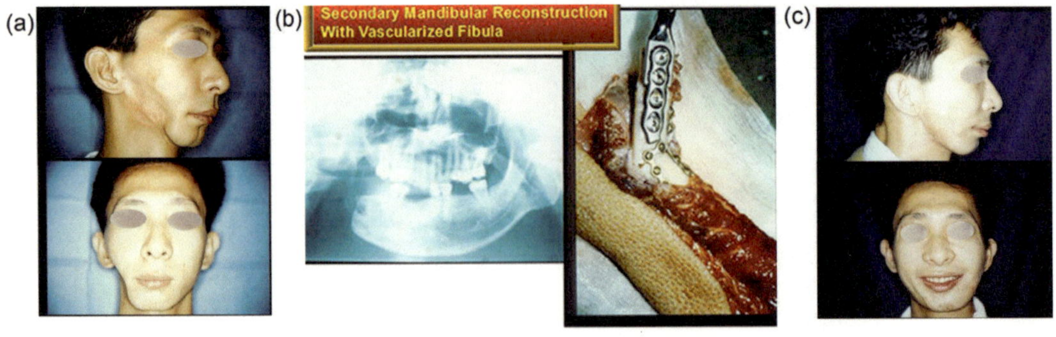

Figure 19. (a) This 27-year-old young man received hemimandibular reconstruction with implant after resection of ameloblastoma, however, complicated with infection and extrusion, ended up with removal of implant, leaving significant facial deformity. (b) The lateral segment mandibular defect was then reconstructed with fibula flap 1 year later. (c) Postoperative photos showing regain of facial contour and symmetricity after reconstruction with fibula flap.

Ancillary procedures:

Ancillary procedures are always required to achieve satisfactory functional and aesthetic results are shown in (**Table 4**) and (**Table 5**).

A. Hemimandibular reconstruction with implant (**Figure 20(a–d)**).

B. Soft tissue wasting above the left mandibular implant area (**Figure 21(a–c)**).

C. Secondary resurfacing of the lower sulcus with a banked iliac bone skin flap with revolving door technique to facilitate denture fitting and restoration of chin profile (**Figure 23(a–f)**).

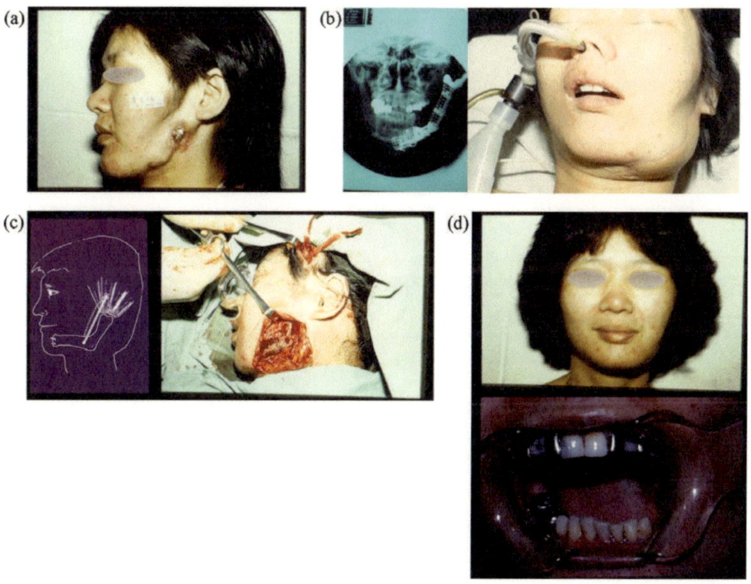

Figure 20. (a) Mandibular implant extrusion with infection. (b) Removal of mandibular implant and reconstruction with vascularized iliac bone flap. Sagging down of the reconstructed mandible was noticed due to lack of holding power of the temporal muscle to coronoid process. (c) Fascial at a sling operation was performed to hold the reconstructed mandible to the temporalis muscle. (d) Post-op front view with adequate mouth opening shown.

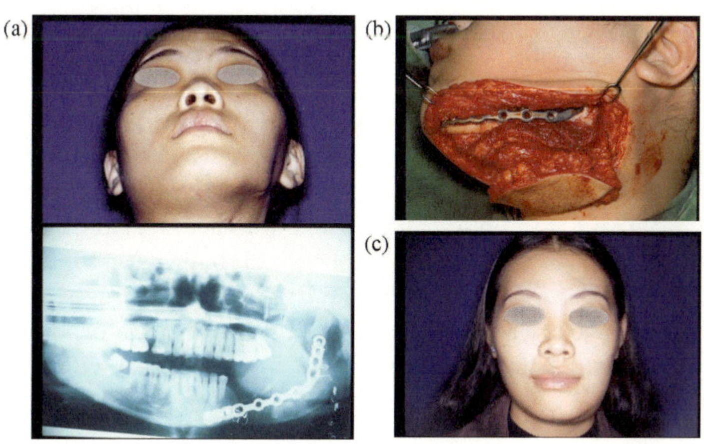

Figure 21. (a) Retention of mandibular implant and onlaying with a vascularized iliac bone flap. (b) Vascularized iliac bone osteocutaneous flap, placed overlying the mandibular implant with osteosynthesis. (c) Postoperative result: soft tissue wasting and atrophy ceased with long term follow up.

Mouth opening
Oral competence
temporo-mandibular joint function
Deepening of buccogingival sulcus
Feasibility in fixation of denture
Osseointegration

Table 4. Functional considerations.

Recontouring of mandibular margin
Soft tissue repositioning
Sliding genioplasty
Fascial sling operation for hemimandibular reconstruction
Myectomy of contralateral lower lip depressors
Z-plasty, W-plasty on scars
Reduction of bulk
Commissuroplasty
Fat graft, fascial graft

Table 5. Aesthetic considerations.

7. Results

In 102 patients presenting with mandibular implant extrusions, the primary etiologies were mostly ameloblastoma (100/102), fibroma (1/102), and malignant mixed tumor (1/102). Before extrusiom of the implant occurs, the implant may be retained and overlaid with a vascularized bone.

Keeping the mandibular implant and overlaying it with a vascularized iliac bone flap can achieve not only a good functional result (**Table 4**) If extrusion of the implant has occurred, infection will supervene, and inevitably the implant should be removed totally. Reconstruction may involve removal of the mandibular implant and immdiate replacement of the mandibular defect with a piece of vascularized bone flap, not only to compensate for bone loss, but also to replace neighboring soft tissue and possible skin defect. With the night strategy, good functional outcome and satisfactory aesthetic result can always be achieved, but also a satisfactory aesthetic outcome (**Table 5**). Soft tissue wasting and atrophy ceased with long-term follow-up (**Figure 22(a)** and **(b)**).

For reconstruction of anterior segment mandibular defect, vascularized iliac bone grafting associated with external banking of the skin and soft tissue, followed by turning the skin flap and soft tissue intraorally with revolving door technique, can resurface the anterior vestibule and augment the chin profile, a procedure that also facilitate fitting lower denture fitting (**Figure 23(a–f)**).

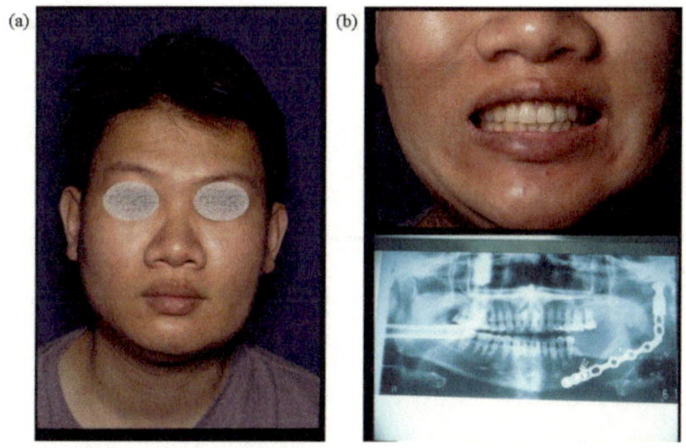

Figure 22. (a) Retention of mandibular implant and overlying with vascularized iliac bone flap can achieve not only good functional result, but also satisfactory aesthetic outcome. (b) Post-op result: soft tissue wasting and atrophy ceased with long-term follow-up.

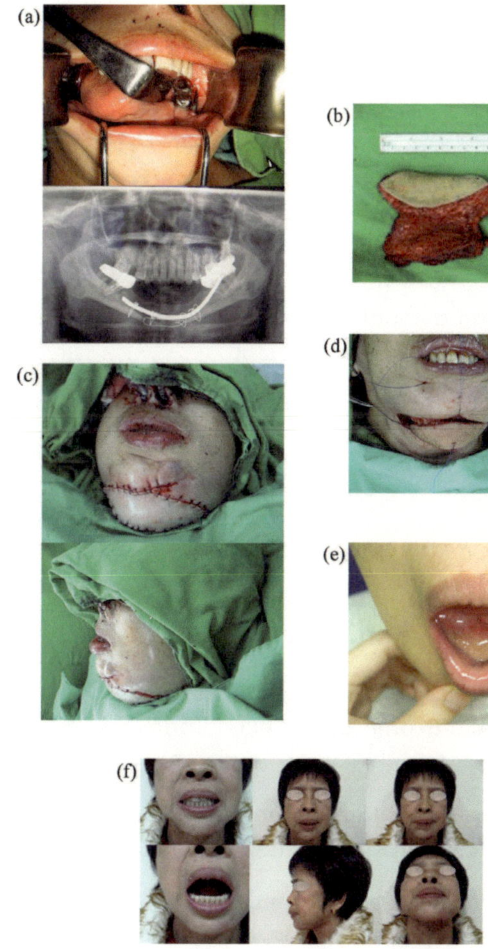

Figure 23. (a) Pre-op. (b) Harvesting of iliac bone osteomyocutaneous flap. (c) Insetting of flap. (d) Flap transposition with revolving door technique. (e) Anterior sulcus reconstruction was completed by employing revolving door technique. (f) Reconstruction of lower sulcus by mobilizing the banked skin flap inward with revolving door technique can accommodate further denture fitting, resulting in good functional and aesthetic result.

8. Discussions

Mandibular defects may result in significant facial disfigurement. When the defect is associated with inner mucosal defect and/or external skin defect, the situation become even more complicated [11]. Conventional bone grafting can only succeed in less than 5 cm segmental defect or partial thickness defect.

Mandibular implants made of different materials (titanium, vitellium, etc.) and having different brands have been used by many head and neck surgeons to reconstruct segmental mandibular defects or hemimandibular defects. However, they are fraught with miscellaneous miserable complications [12].

In this article, we have presented many kinds of failures resulting from mandibular reconstructions with implants.

Reconstructions problems associated with implant failure include:

- scarring and capsule formation around the implant,
- difficulty in dissecting and approaching the glenoid fossa,
- lack of a clear plane to expand the pocket in order to accommodate a vascularized bone graft camouflaging the ascending ramus, resulting in
- possibility of facial nerve injury or traction during dissection or expansion.
- Careful planning of the incision should be elaborated because of soft tissue atrophy and thinning of skin on top of the mandibular implant.

The choice of bone flap for reconstructions is iliac bone flap for anterior mandibular, segmental and hemimandibular reconstructions while, for lateral mandibular defect, fibular flap in preferred.

9. Conclusions

The fate of various reconstructive modes for major mandibular defects has been presented. Selecting the ideal modes of reconstruction for significant mandibular defects is of paramount importance if an uncomplicated outcome and excellent functional result without facial disfigurement are to be achieved.

Secondary mandibular reconstruction after implant failure may cause facial nerve injury due to scarring which result in difficulty in approaching the glenoid fossa.

When mandibular reconstruction with implant fails, extrusion and infection may ensue and necessitate removal of the implant. In this situation, soft tissue wasting, fibrosis, and contracture will supervene. The overlying facial nerve will be endangered during further reconstruction consequent upon creating additional space to accommodate a vascularized bone flap.

A fascia lata sling operation is always required in hemimandibular reconstruction in patients with the implant failures, in order to hold the reconstructed mandible to an anatomical and functional place.

The use of mandibular implants as the sole reconstruction tool for significant mandibular defects should be limited. Since patients suffering from mandibular ameloblastomas are mostly young, it is advised that vascularized bone be the ideal choice in major mandibular reconstructions.

Acknowledgements

The authors are indebted to Ms. Hsiao-Fang Wei and Ms. Fang-I Chu for their assistance in preparing and finishing this manuscript. Without their endeavor, this chapter would not come out so soon.

Author details

Shih-Heng Chen[1,2], Hao-Chih Tai[2], Tai-Ju Cheng[2], Hung-Chi Chen[3], An-Ta Ko[4], Tyng-Luan Roan[4], Yo-Shen Chen[4] and Yueh-Bih Tang[2,4*]

*Address all correspondence to: phoebetang0103@gmail.com

1 Chang-Gung Memorial Hospital, Taoyuan, Taiwan

2 National Taiwan University Hospital, Taipei, Taiwan

3 China Medical University Hospital, Taichung City, Taiwan

4 Far-Eastern Memorial Hospital, New Taipei City, Taiwan

References

[1] Hidalgo DA. Deep circumflex iliac artery free flaps. In: Shaw WW, Hidalgo DA, editors. Microsurgery in Trauma. Mount Kisco, New York: Futura Publishing Company, Inc; 1988

[2] Chen YB, Chen HC, Hahn LH. Major mandibular reconstruction with vascularized bone grafts: Indications and selection of donor tissue. Microsurgery. 1994;**15**(4):227-237

[3] Boyd JB. Use of reconstruction plates in conjunction with soft-tissue free flaps for oromandibular reconstruction. Clinics in Plastic Surgery. 1994;**21**(1):69-77

[4] Hidalgo DA. Aesthetic improvements in free-flap mandible reconstruction. Plastic and Reconstructive Surgery. 1991;**88**(4):574-585; discussion 586-587

[5] Roan TL, et al. New modified free chimeric fibular flap design for head and neck reconstruction. Head & Neck. 2013;**35**(8):E231-E233

[6] Boyd JB. The place of the iliac crest in vascularized oromandibular reconstruction. Microsurgery. 1994;**15**(4):250-256

[7] Chen SH, et al. Reconstruction for osteoradionecrosis of the mandible: Superiority of free iliac bone flap to fibula flap in postoperative infection and healing. Annals of Plastic Surgery. 2014;**73**(Suppl 1):S18-S26

[8] Taylor GI. Reconstruction of the mandible with free composite iliac bone grafts. Annals of Plastic Surgery. 1982;**9**(5):361-376

[9] Taylor GI, Townsend P, Corlett R. Superiority of the deep circumflex iliac vessels as the supply for free groin flaps. Plastic and Reconstructive Surgery. 1979;**64**(5):595-604

[10] Chen YB, Chen SH, Chen HC. Finesse in Aesthetic Facial Recontouring. Oral Cancer, InTech Open Science, Croatia, 2012

[11] Chen SH, et al. Features of oral cancers in Taiwanese females with free tissue transfers: Based on NTUH data. Plastic and Reconstructive Surgery R.O.C. 2009;**18**(4):311-320

[12] Chen YB, Hahn LJ, Yao YT. Long-term survival of patients with mandibular osteosarcoma. Journal of the Formosan Medical Association. 1999;**98**(11):773-777

Chapter 7

Hand Coverage

Francisco Martinez Martinez,
M. Llanos Guerrero Navarro, Juan Garcia Navarro,
Alberto Gimenez Ros and
Alba Izquierdo Robledano

Additional information is available at the end of the chapter

http://dx.doi.org/10.5772/intechopen.74152

Abstract

Hand and finger soft tissue defects have always represented a surgical challenge at any accident and emergency department. Techniques may vary from just direct closure of the wound to free tissue transfer. Knowledge of the main locoregional hand flaps is paramount to solve most of the soft tissue defects at this level. Flaps vary depending on their blood supply and design. Their vascularity might be at random, they can be pedicled with anterograde or reversed flow or they can rely on simple or complex free tissue transfer whose blood flow depends on vascular anastomosis. This article reviews all the main soft tissue local or locoregional reconstructive techniques for hands and fingers.

Keywords: hand coverage, hand reconstruction, fingertip reconstruction, soft tissue defect

1. Introduction

Soft tissue coverage represents an essential part of the treatment of a traumatic hand. Conservative approach of soft tissue loss may lead to irreversible stiffness and in some cases a higher chance of infection.

The design of different flaps for the hand has been the result of an improvement in the knowledge of hand neurovascular anatomy as well as their hemodynamic behaviour. This has allowed the development of an immense variety of regional flaps to fit a wide range of soft tissue problems.

Before all this knowledge, flaps were harvested at random, and a 2:1 width to length relation was a necessary condition in order to ensure the survival of a flap. This represented an important limitation to solve the different soft tissue challenges.

The description of pedicled flaps importantly increased the possibilities of coverage. The first neurovascular pedicled island flap was described by Littler [1]. Reverse-flow pedicled flap was first described by Foucher [3] based on the distal anastomotic connections with the dorsal metacarpal arteries, which were found in anatomy studies. Besides, the later description of perforator flaps also simplified the reconstructive techniques, avoiding the sacrifice of important vascular structures. Pollicisation of the index finger, already performed in congenital hand cases, was also applied in traumatic loss of the thumb. Eventually, the development of microsurgical advanced techniques such as toe to finger transfer for partial or complete amputation of a finger was an important asset in cosmesis and function.

Currently, our effort has also been focused not merely on coverage but also on reducing donor site morbidity; techniques leading to incapacitating neuralgias or scars have to be avoided. In some patients, this type of pain may represent a more serious problem than stiffness itself.

There are different possibilities of coverage depending on the tissue exposed and its location. This chapter will only deal with locoregional basic flaps.

2. Split- and full-thickness skin grafts

This type of technique (**Figure 1**) can only be used when bones or tendons are not exposed. Due to inevitable contracture after the graft has taken, most patients will need some sort of

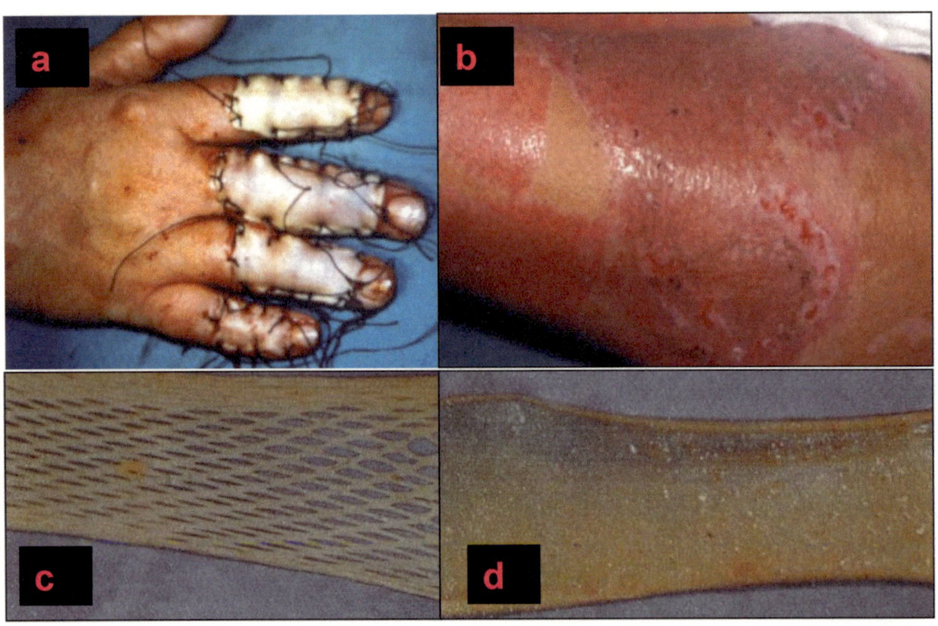

Figure 1. Skin grafts: (a) full-thickness skin grafts applied to the dorsum of the hands, (b) donor site of split-thickness skin grafts, (c) split-thickness skin graft meshed and (d) split-thickness skin graft.

hand physiotherapy. This is even more the case, when partial-thickness skin grafts have been used. This type of graft is more prone to contract after having taken.

Split-thickness skin grafts have to be harvested with the help of a dermatome and must be 0.25–0.3 mm wide. Thicker grafts may lead to a non-healing donor site plus a less chance of graft taking. They are often meshed in order to increase their size and to allow exudate to escape.

Full-thickness skin grafts are usually used in finger coverage. One of the reasons is that the amount of the skin to cover a defect in fingers is small enough to be easily obtained from the groin, the wrist or even the anterior skin of the arm or forearm. Also, this type of graft tends to contract less that the split one allows a better functional and cosmetic result.

3. Local flaps for the dorsum of the hand

The dorsal skin of the hand is particularly elastic, and different local flaps can be performed in order to cover small defects. The blood supply is mostly at random in these flaps. They might be useful when small to moderate defects are approached and mostly if bone or tendons are exposed. The palmar skin of the hand can be considered the opposite in these terms. Local flaps will not usually solve any coverage difficulty.

Cuadrangular skin advancements and rotational flaps are simple and allow stable coverage with optimal rates of survival.

Limberg or Dufourmentel (**Figure 2**) flaps are local cuadrangular transposition flaps. These are mostly performed in elective surgery such as excisional removal of lesions [2].

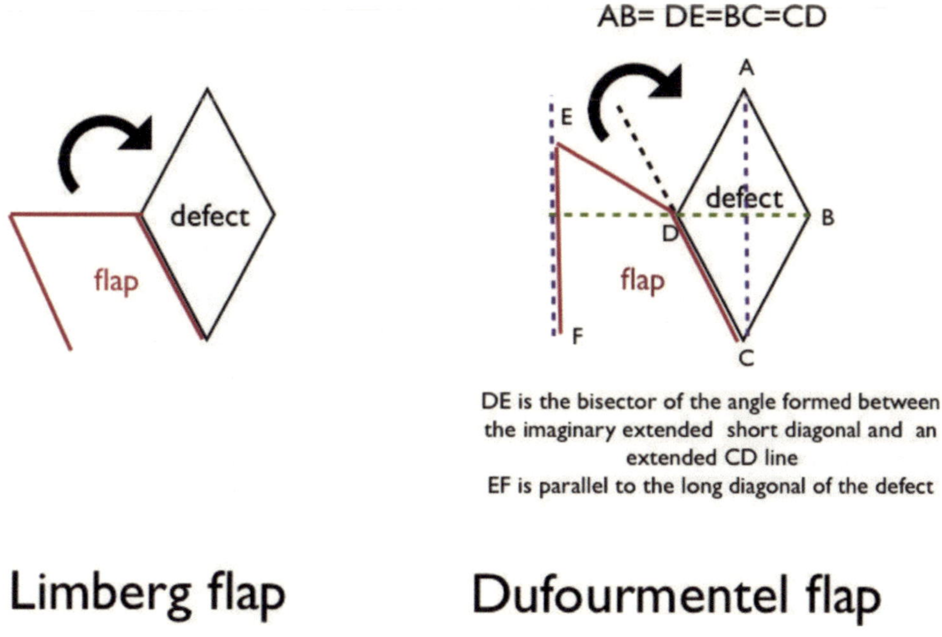

Figure 2. Limberg's and Dufourmentel's flaps.

4. Coverage of the palm of the hand

4.1. Radial fasciocutaneous flap

Described by Yang [4] in 1981 as a free flap for the hand, this is a fasciocutaneous island flap based on the radial artery. Currently, it is not considered the first surgical option due to inevitable sacrifice of the radial artery and possible donor site morbidity. Allen's test is performed before surgical planning (**Figure 3**).

When the objective is palm coverage, the design of the paddle starts in the middle third of the forearm between the brachioradialis (BR) and the flexor carpi radialis (FCR). The dissection can be performed suprafascially, but once the septum in between the two muscles is reached, the fascia along with the septum and the artery has to be included. The peritenons of the FCR and BR must not be injured. The cephalic vein is usually necessary when harvesting a free flap but not in the case of a reverse-flow type, in which only concomitant veins are needed. The artery will be ligated at the proximal aspect of the flap. The arterial blood flow to the radial artery occurs through the distal ulnar artery connections in the vascular palmar arches; thus, this will then be considered a reverse-flow island flap.

The same flap can also be raised as an adipofascial flap in order to reduce morbidity of the donor site, but then again the flap itself will have to be grafted. An osteocutaneous radial flap

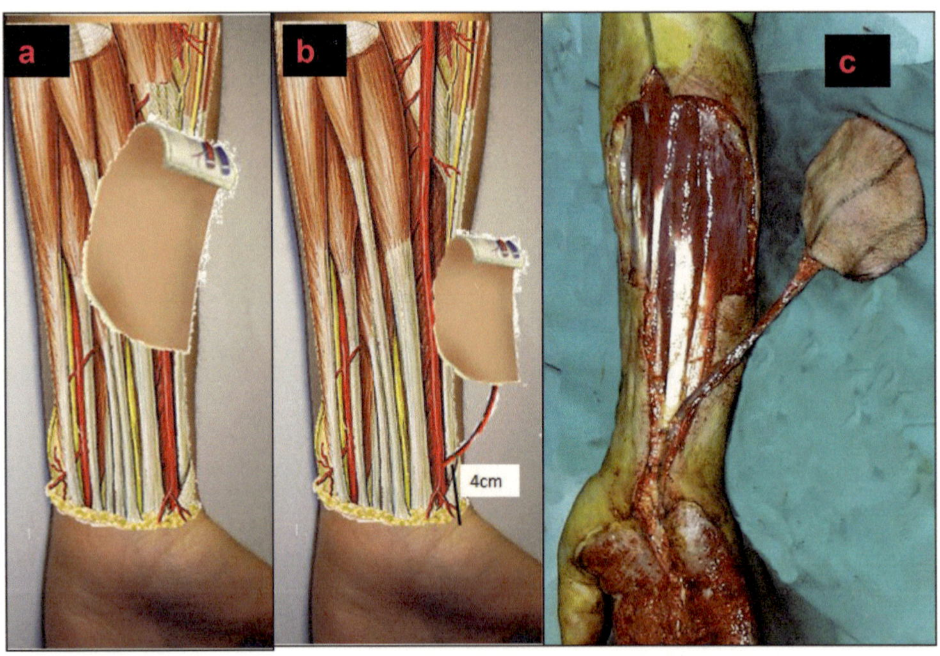

Figure 3. Fasciocutaneous radial flap: (a) retrograde fasciocutaneous radial flap, (b) radial perforator flap and (c) clinical case of a retrograde fasciocutaneous radial flap for a defect of the palm of the hand.

has also been described. In this case a small portion of the radius diaphysis is taken along with the artery. This type of reconstruction has been widely used as a free flap and not much as a pedicled flap.

A perforator radial flap has also been described based on about ten existent perforating vessels (0.3–0.5 mm in diameter) located 2–4 cm proximal to the radial styloid process. To raise an adipofasciocutaneous flap, the territory will be marked over the proximal or middle third of the volar aspect of the forearm, with the pivot point about 2–4 cm proximal to the radial styloid. The proximal perforators can be ligated leaving the distal ones intact. The flap can be also potentially raised as an adipofascial flap [5].

4.2. Glabrous skin flap

Orbay et al. [6] described a flap based on a superficial cutaneous branch of the radial artery at the thenar eminence (**Figure 4**).

The superficial palmar arch is mainly formed by the ulnar artery, less so the superficial branch of the radial artery emerges 1–2 cm proximal to the wrist fold before dividing into superficial and dorsal branches (the latter one eventually enters Guyon's canal).

The superficial radial branch courses underneath the palmar fascia and irrigates the thenar eminence before proceeding under the adductor and opponens muscles. At the level of the insertion of the FCR, the cutaneous branch of the superficial radial artery perforates the palmar

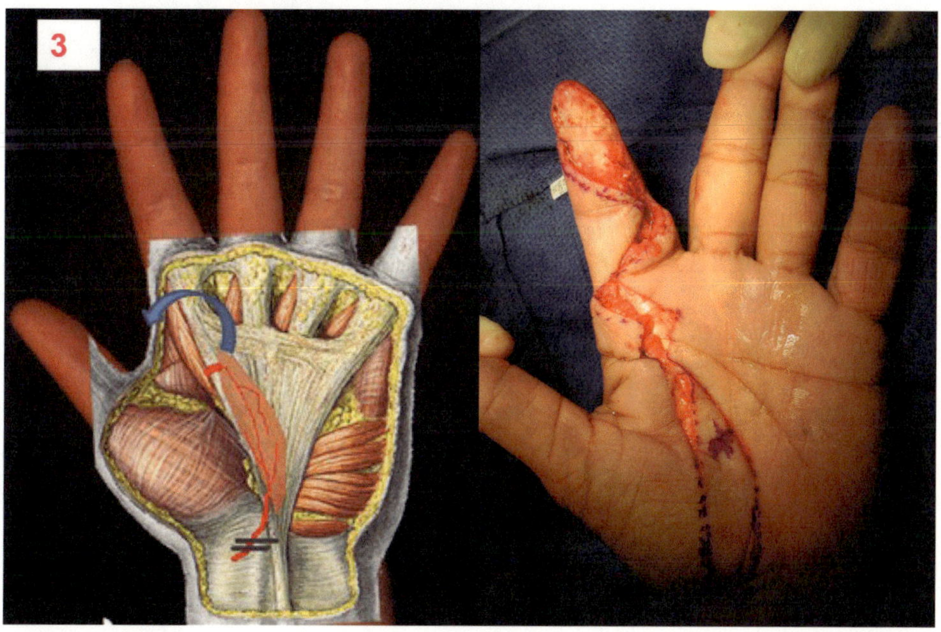

Figure 4. Reverse-flow flap based on the anastomosis of the superficial palmar branch of the radial artery with the vascular palmar arches. Notice the 180° arc of rotation of the flap.

fascia; this level corresponds to a point 0.5–1 cm radial to the cutaneous thenar fold. A distal perforating vessel from the profundus or the superficial arch emerges at the confluency of Kaplan's line with the second webspace axis. The flap can then be raised based on the proximal cutaneous perforator and down to the radial superficial artery. Thus raised, the flap can be used as a free flap. Based on the distal perforators, it can also be designed to be a retrograde flap and can be used to solve first web contractures. In this case the superficial radial branch must be ligated proximal to the skin paddle.

5. Coverage of the dorsum of the hand

5.1. Posterior interosseous fasciocutaneous flap

Described by Zancolli and Angrigiani [7] in 1988 for the dorsal coverage of the hand, this flap is based on the existence of an anastomosis between the posterior interosseous artery and the dorsal branch of the anterior interosseous artery at the dorsal aspect of the wrist. The posterior interosseous artery will be ligated, and the blood flow will course retrogradely from the anterior interosseous artery to the posterior interosseous pedicle (**Figure 5**).

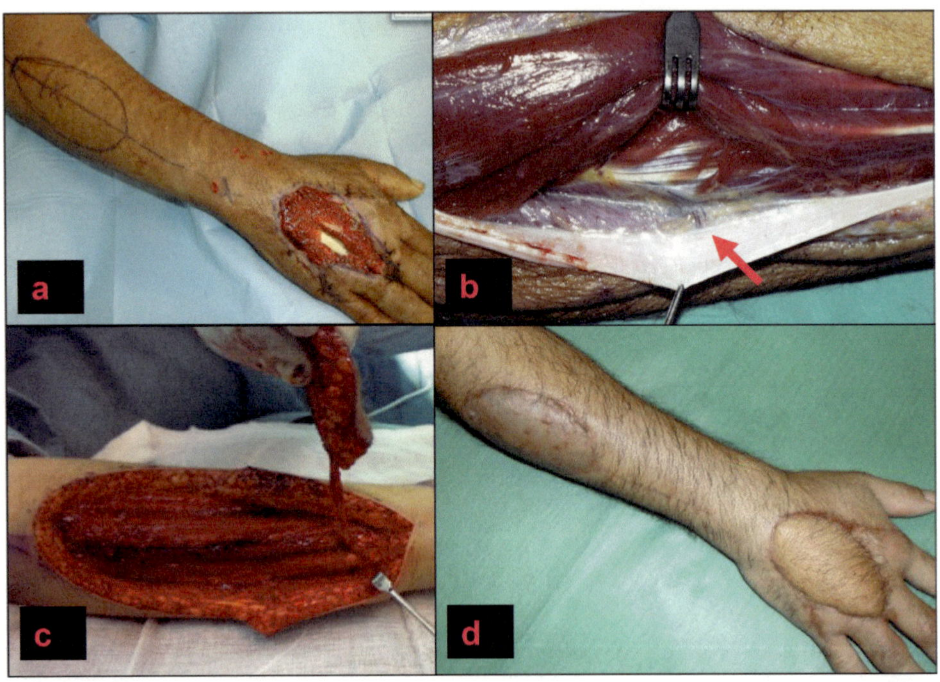

Figure 5. Interosseous posterior flap: (a) defect located on the dorsum of the hand and markings of the flap, (b) septum between the fifth and sixth extensor compartment where a cutaneous perforator can be visualized, (c) the flap harvested and (d) the final outcome.

http://dx.doi.org/10.5772/intechopen.74152

The design of the posterior interosseous flap starts with the marking of the cutaneous island. A line is drawn between the lateral humeral epicondyle and the distal radioulnar joint. The island must be outlined in between the proximal and distal thirds of the forearm. The main posterior interosseous cutaneous branch emerges 9 centimetres distal to the lateral epicondyle in the same line; this can also be easily identified with a Doppler ultrasound.

The vascular anastomosis between the two interosseous arteries can be found 2 cm proximal to the radiocarpal joint at the proximal border of the pronator quadratus.

The interosseous posterior artery is found at the septum between the extensor carpi ulnaris (ECU) and the extensor digiti minimi (EDM). This septum and the anastomosis are easily identified distally, which is the reason why many surgeons prefer to first identify the anastomosis and the posterior interosseous artery and eventually raise the flap. The posterior interosseous artery is closely related with the posterior interosseous nerve. This condition might represent a challenge in the hands of an inexperienced surgeon.

Donor site may be close directly or with a split skin graft depending on the width of the cutaneous island.

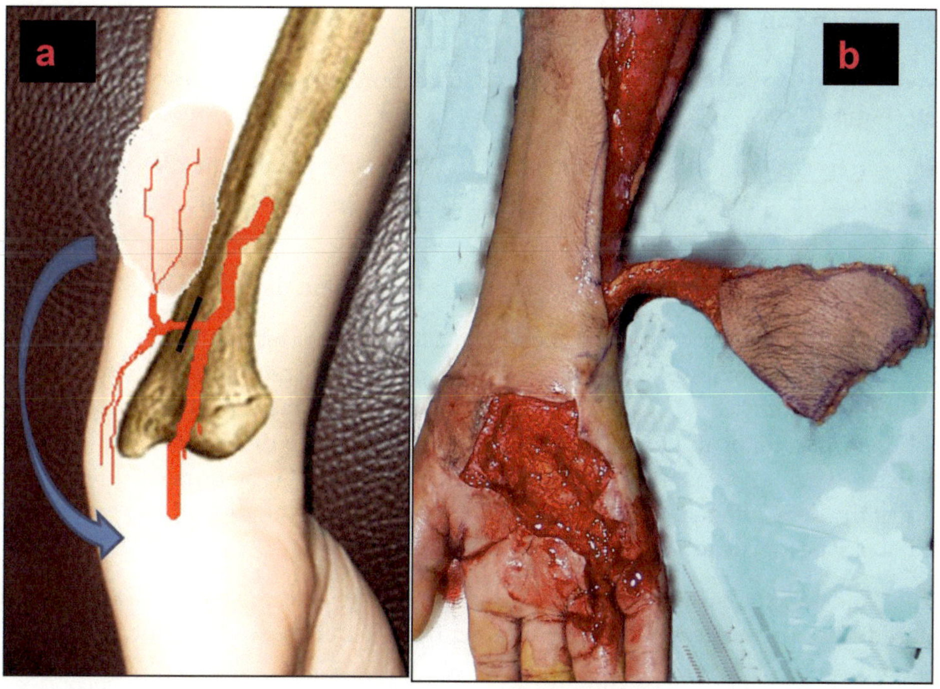

Figure 6. Dorsoulnar fasciocutaneous flap: (a) anatomy of the distal dorsal branch of the ulnar artery and elevation of the flap based on the distal anastomosis of the ascending branch with the dorsal radial arch and the cutaneous ulnar branch needs to be ligated in order to perform a retrograde flap (black line) and (b) clinical case of dorsoulnar fasciocutaneous flap to cover a defect of the palm.

5.2. Dorsoulnar fasciocutaneous flap

This is a flap that is based on the distal branch of the ulnar artery which emerges 2–5 cm proximal to the pisiform bone. This branch courses between the flexor carpi ulnaris (FCU) and the ECU and then reaches the cutaneous skin crossing between the ulnar nerve and the FCU distally. It then divides into descending and ascending branches. The descending branch anastomoses with skin perforators of the dorsal arch (**Figure 6**).

This distal branch can be identified with Doppler ultrasound. The flap can then be raised as a propeller flap (rotating the fasciocutaneous island around this branch) or as a reversed flap based on the anastomosis with the descending branch. This second option allows further advancement. This flap reaches the fourth and the fifth metacarpophalangeal joints.

Bertelli and Pagliei [8] have made an anatomic description of an osteocutaneous flap based on the ulnar periosteal branches of the ascending branch.

6. Finger coverage

6.1. Cross-finger flap

The cross-finger flap is a two-stage flap reconstruction that was first described by Cronin in 1951 [9] (**Figure 7**).

This flap can be easily raised due to the fact that it does not require the dissection of vascular pedicles. It is a transposition flap based on the subcutaneous dorsal branches of a proper palm digital artery (PDA).

The fact that this is a two-stage surgical technique is the main disadvantage.

This flap is frequently designed over the dorsal skin of a medial phalanx in order to cover a distal phalanx or a medial phalanx of a contiguous finger. The limits of flap dissection are always represented by the finger folds. The vascular base of the flap is located at the mediolateral line of the donor finger that is directly opposite to the defect on the adjacent finger. In the case of volar skin loss, the flap has to be raised based on the dorsal skin of the medial phalanx of the donor finger. In case of dorsal skin loss, the coverage will be performed based on the volar aspect instead.

Dissection must include the skin and subcutaneous tissue, and the tendon sheath should not be exposed. The donor site has to be covered with a full-thickness skin graft.

The donor and recipient finger should be buddy splinted for 2 weeks. The second surgical step is then performed and the syndactyly is released. Hand physiotherapy will be necessary after the surgical procedure has been completed.

This type of coverage is particularly interesting for the triphalangeal fingers. The middle finger acts as a proper donor for the index and ring fingers. Little finger injuries require the skin

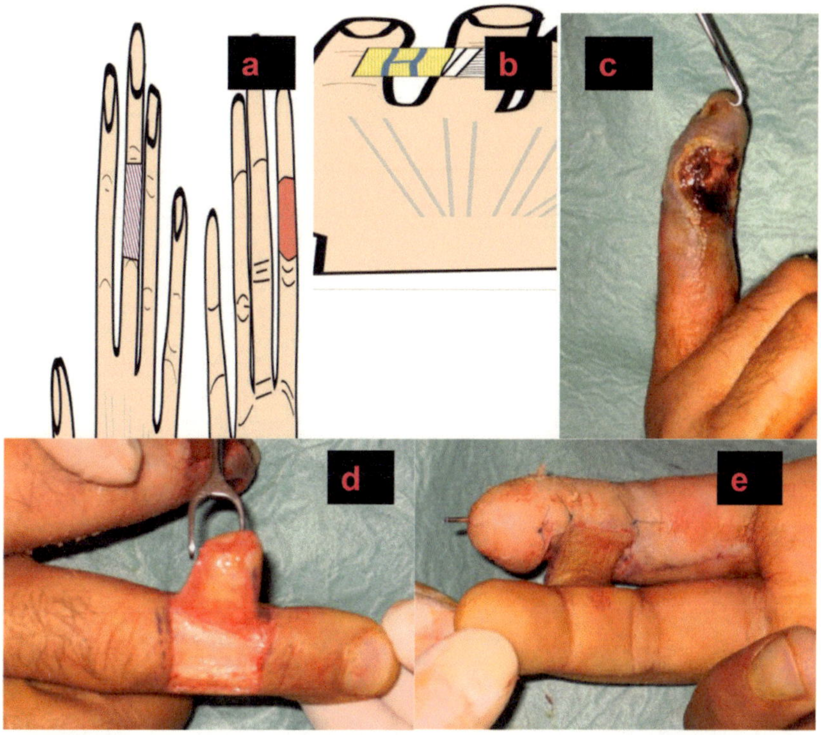

Figure 7. Cross-finger flap: (a and b) defect and markings of the flap and (c, d and e) clinical case; always preserve the peritenon to be able to apply a skin graft on the donor digit.

from the ring finger. This flap is not a good option for the coverage of the tip of the middle finger, because the ring or the index medial phalanges are more proximally located and the middle finger needs to be forced into flexion in order to fit next to them.

6.2. Thenar flap

This flap has also been described for the reconstruction of the tip of the long fingers. This is not only a simple technique but also needs a two-step procedure (**Figure 8**).

The skin is taken from the radial aspect of the thenar eminence, proximal to the metacarpo-phalangeal fold. Despite of its name, scars at the thenar eminence should be avoided above all the weight-bearing central axis of the thenar eminence.

The base of the flap can be cranially or caudally located. The donor site needs to be grafted.

6.3. V to Y Atasoy flap

This triangular advancement flap was described by Tranquili [10] and popularised by Atasoy [11]. This flap is indicated in the case of transverse or dorsally oblique amputation of the tip of the fingers (**Figure 9a**).

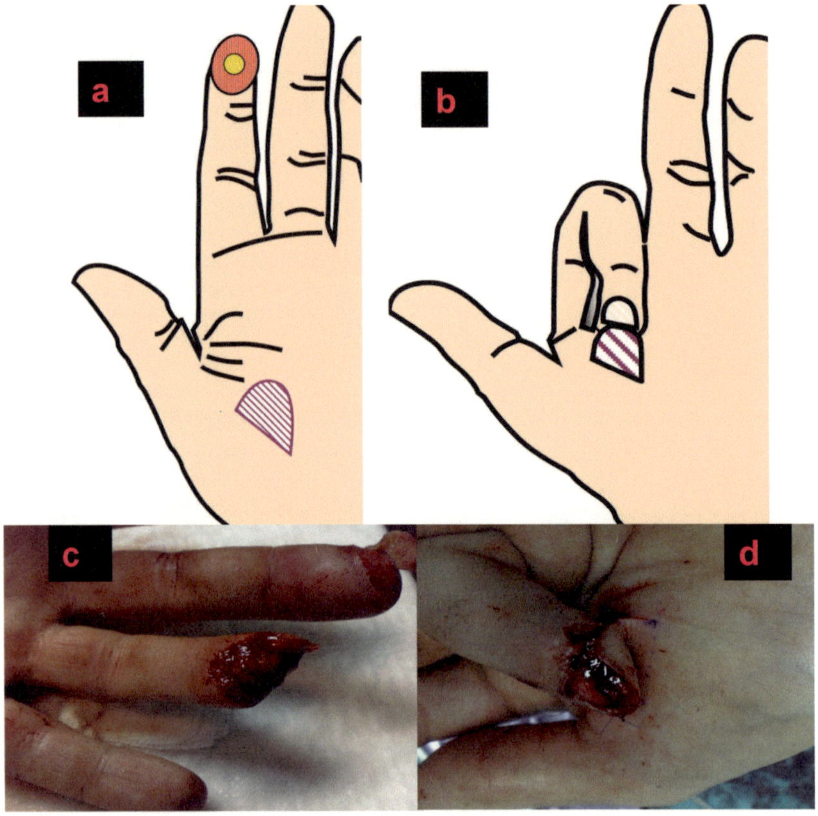

Figure 8. Thenar flap: (a and b) schema and (c and d) clinical case.

This flap is one of the most frequently performed in the emergency department but can be advanced only up to 7 to 8 mms. If higher expectations are sought, this flap would not be suitable. Inexperienced surgeons may tend to skeletonize the base of the flap or suture it under tension; any of these situations lead to inevitable flap necrosis.

The design of the flap is marked on the volar aspect of the affected distal phalanx down to the distal fold. The subcutaneous tissue can be fully elevated from the tendon sheath. The skin will only be incised superficially (i.e. until the subcutaneous tissue appears). Once dissected, the distal aspect of the flap is fixed with the help of a small needle rather than direct sutures, because direct suturing may damage the nail bed. The skin must be closed in a V to Y fashion in order to advance the flap.

6.4. Bilateral V to Y Kutler's flap

This bilateral flap was described by Kutler [12] in 1930; it is based on the same principles as the V to Y flap (**Figure 9b**).

The Vs are marked at both sides of the defect, taking into account that they will be irrigated by the small branches of the proper palmar digital arteries.

http://dx.doi.org/10.5772/intechopen.74152

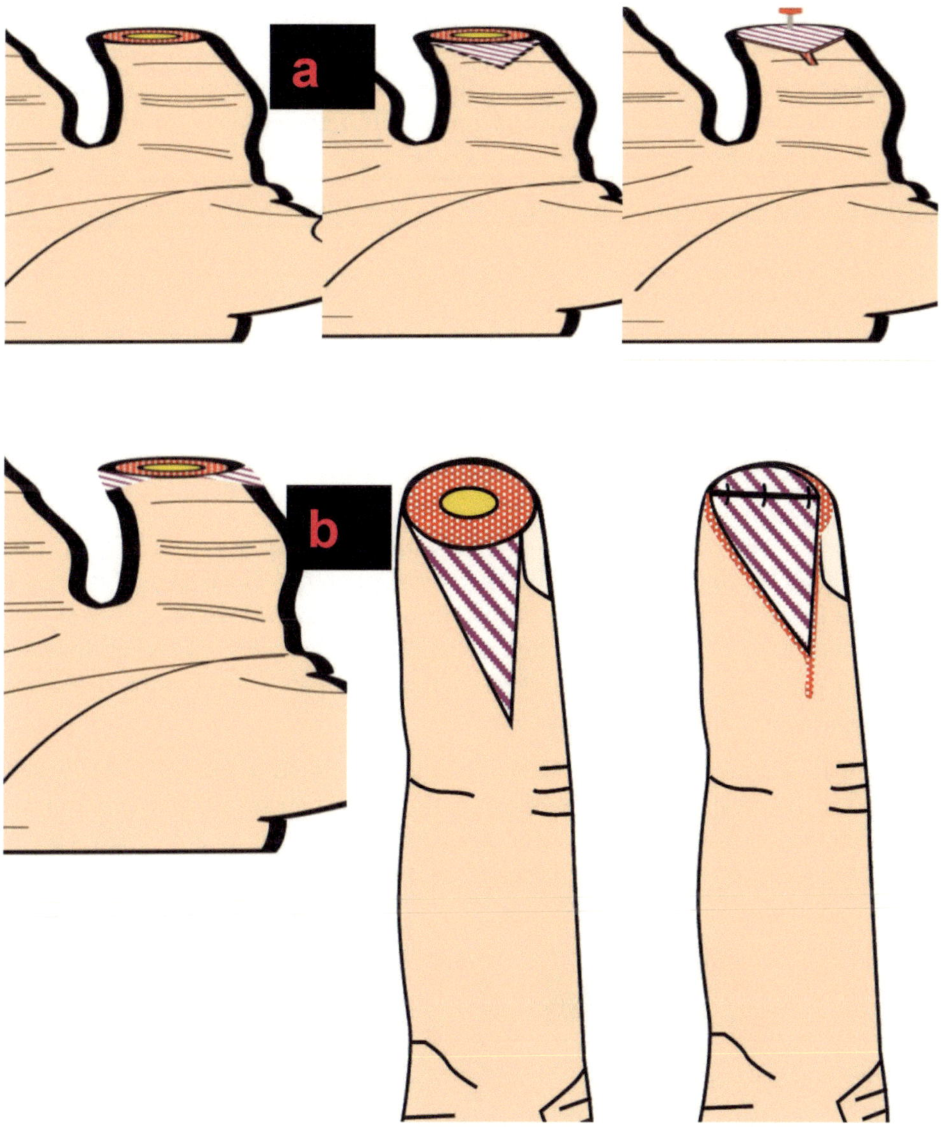

Figure 9. (a) Atasoy's flap and (b) Kutler's flap.

As a main drawback, this flap leaves an unpleasant longitudinal linear scar at the tip of the finger.

6.5. Homodigital pedicled island flaps

6.5.1. Oblique triangular neurovascular flap

This flap was described by Venkataswami and Subramanian [13] in 1980; it is mostly suitable for oblique fingertip amputations. The flap is based on the vascular pedicle opposite the amputated side. The base of the triangular flap lies adjacent to de amputated side. A vertical incision is performed in the midlateral line of the finger down to the periosteum, and the pedicle of the finger is visualised and fully raised avoiding skeletonization. A partial thickness oblique incision is then performed; only the fibrous septa are divided to allow flap advancement (**Figure 10**).

The apex of the triangle is usually marked at the PIP joint. Small islands will tend to contract in time. Therefore, the island should never be small in size.

Unlike most unipedicled digital flaps, it contains the digital nerve of the flap and branches of the contralateral digital nerve. It cannot be considered as a true island flap but the first step just before that.

In case the advancement provided is insufficient, decision has to be made as to whether a true island flap is needed.

6.5.2. Homodigital neurovascular anterograde unipedicled island flap

This was described by Littler [1] although as a heterodigital flap. The design of the flap is subject to the location of the lesion. Despite of that, Brunelli described some considerations as to which donor site is more advisable in order to leave intact the dominant hemipulp. Advisable donor sites are the ulnar aspect of the index and middle fingers as well as the radial aspect of the ring and little fingers (**Figures 11** and **12**).

A U-shaped flap is marked, proximal to the defect, apex based at the PIP joint. The vertical incision reaches the periosteum, and once again, the pedicle must be visualised and not skeletonized to preserve a suitable venous drainage. The oblique incision also reaches the tendon sheath, and the flap would finally only be attached by its pedicle. The advancement can be

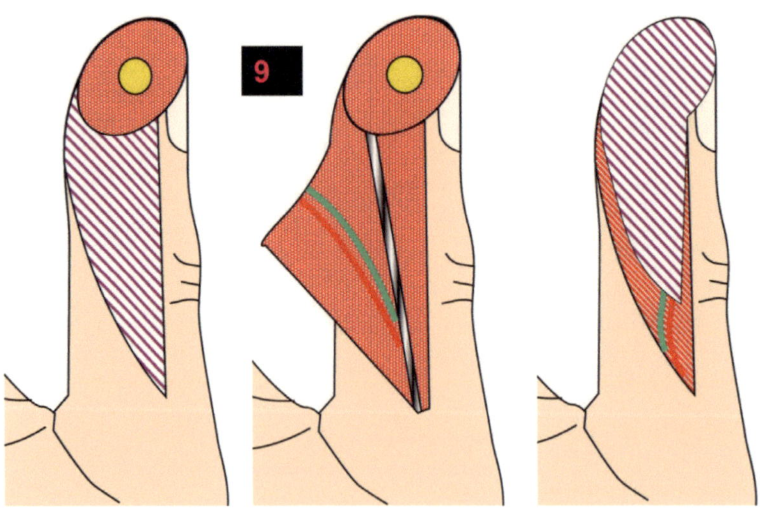

Figure 10. Neurovascular island flap and Venkataswami's flap.

http://dx.doi.org/10.5772/intechopen.74152

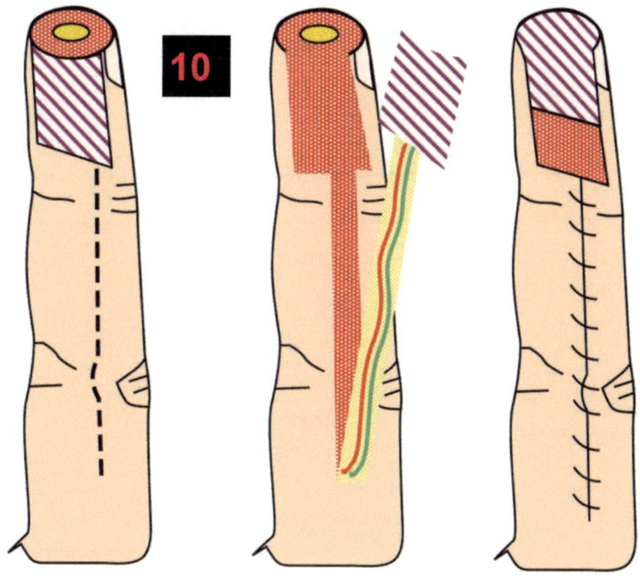

Figure 11. Homodigital anterograde neurovascular flap.

improved by releasing the pedicle down to the base of the finger. Brunner or hemi-Brunner incisions are then performed to avoid scar contractures in the future.

A full-thickness skin graft is hardly ever necessary to cover the donor site.

A splint is advisable in the first week to prevent tension of the pedicle; the MCP joints should be kept flexed and the DIP and PIP joints extended. Hand physiotherapy is paramount to fully recover function.

This flap is not suitable for patients with peripheral vascular disease or in digits nourished by a single vessel.

6.5.3. Homodigital quadrangular flap

Described in 1966 by Hueston [14], this flap is meant to be advanced and rotated to reach the defect. It is based on one of the neurovascular pedicles and is eligible for transverse defects. Further dissection of the pedicle down to the base of the finger is not performed (**Figures 13** and **14**).

The island paddle is outlined at the midaxial lateral line of the less affected side, or in case of a complete transverse amputation, the lateral line transected will correspond to the nondominant side. Therefore, this flap will be based on the dominant neurovascular pedicle. The flap is elevated and the tendon sheath will be left intact. The flap will then be advanced and rotated to cover the area of defect.

The proximal end will be closed in a V to Y fashion or with a skin graft if needed.

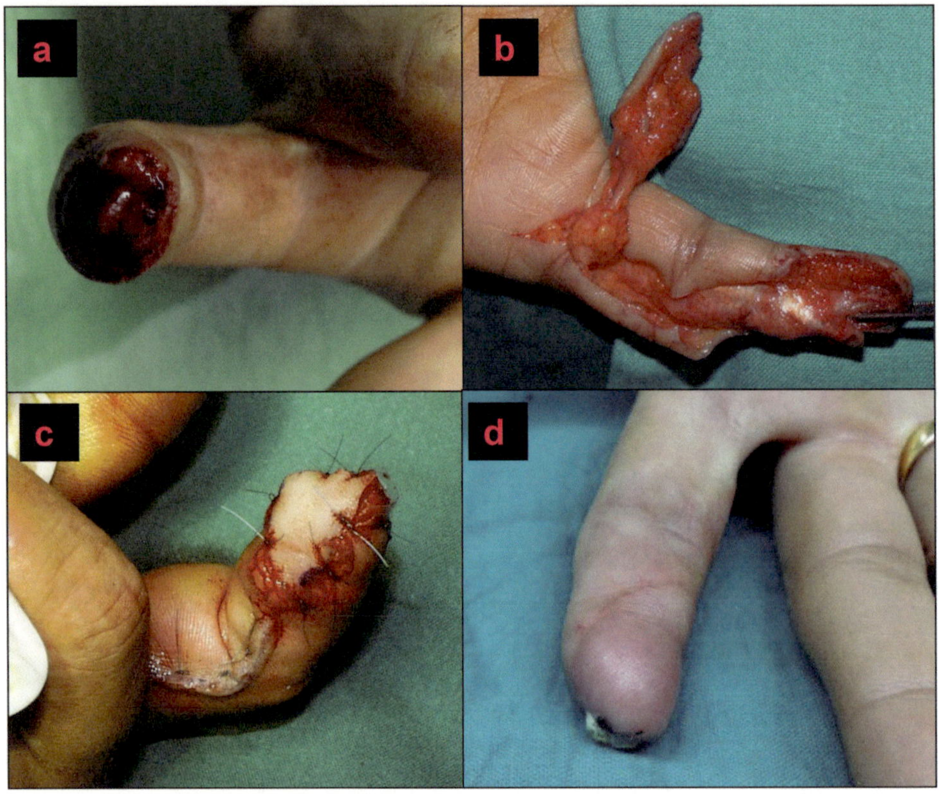

Figure 12. Clinical case of a homodigital anterograde neurovascular flap: (a) distal amputation, (b) flap dissection, (c) result at the end of the surgery and (d) the final outcome.

6.5.4. Homodigital neurovascular retrograde unipedicled flap

Described by Lai [15] in 1989, this flap is outlined on the lateral nondominant border of the base of the affected digit. The availability of the skin paddle is larger than the one for the anterograde flap (**Figure 15**).

Elevation is carried out from proximal to distal until enough length of the pedicle is obtained. The vascularity of this flap is dependent on transverse commissural arteries found at the PIP and DIP joints. Therefore, dissection should not proceed more than 1 cm proximal to the DIP joint. During dissection the proper digital nerve (PDN) is gently separated from the vascular pedicle, and the digital vessel is ligated proximally. The artery must be raised along with a cuff of fat and again never skeletonised the pedicle.

A full-thickness skin graft is used to close the secondary defect at the donor site.

The flap described is a non-sensate flap, and the PDN is left buried under a skin graft, which in some cases may be the cause of scar donor site dysaesthesias.

A retrograde sensate flap has also been described, including the PDN along with the artery. Once the flap reaches the defect, the nerve needs to be sutured to the amputated contralateral nerve in order to achieve sensation.

http://dx.doi.org/10.5772/intechopen.74152

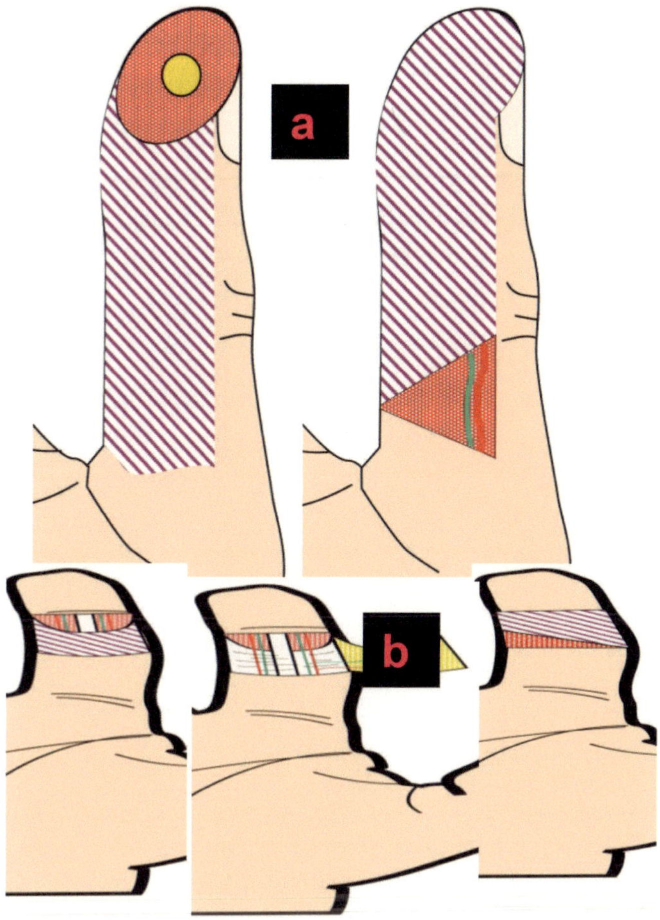

Figure 13. Hueston's flap: (a) schema of the flap for a thumb defect and (b) schema of the flap for a triphalangeal finger.

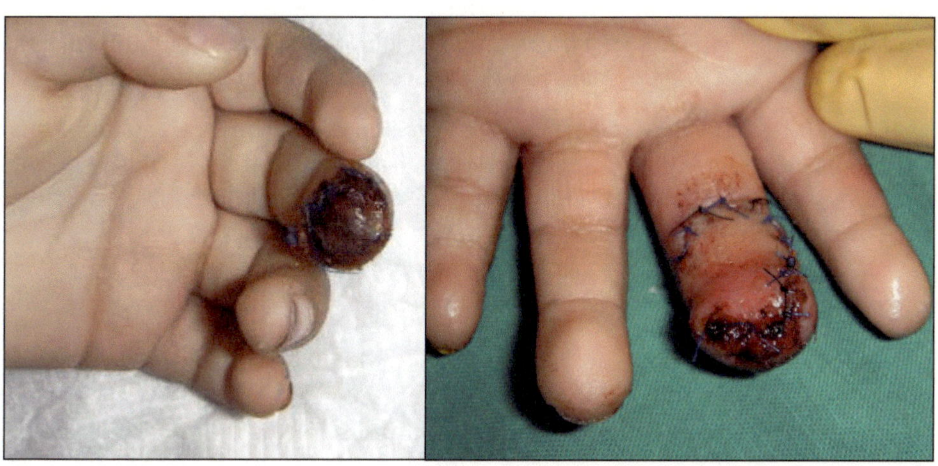

Figure 14. Clinical case of homodigital cuadrangular flap after necrosis of the tip of the middle finger.

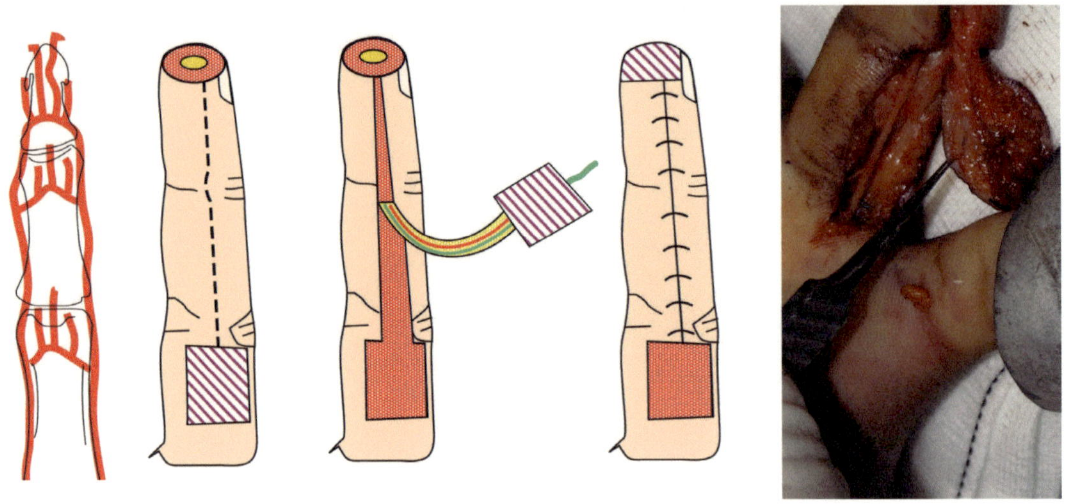

Figure 15. Homodigital retrograde neurovascular flap. The vascular conections of the proper palmar digital arteries are represented on the left image.

The main drawback is the fact that the stump of the donor nerve might turn into a neuroma and neuralgic pain may be quite invalidating.

6.5.5. Homodigital bipedicled island flap for the thumb

Moberg [16] first described this flap in 1964, which consisted of undermining of the volar skin from the dorsal aspect along the midaxial lines of the thumb, starting proximal to the defect. The quadrangular advancement of the volar skin includes the two proper digital arteries and nerves. The arterial supply of the thumb differs from other fingers. Whereas the volar side of the thumb is supplied by two palmar collateral arteries which are branches of the princeps pollicis artery, the dorsal skin is predominantly supplied by ulnar and radial dorsolateral arteries and branches of the dorsal branch of the radial artery. Due to this particular vascularity, this flap can be raised to cover distal defects of the thumb but can potentially cause dorsal skin necrosis in triphalangeal fingers. The IP joint of the thumb should be kept flexed at 15–20° for a week, and later on hand physiotherapy is advised (**Figure 16**).

O'Brien [17] modified this flap in order to avoid flexion contractures. He added a skin incision distal to the MCP fold. Both pedicles are visualised and left intact with surrounding the subcutaneous tissue. This technique allows further advancement of the flap. A graft is then placed to cover this secondary defect.

6.5.6. Homodigital unipedicle retrograde island flap for the thumb

This flap was described by Brunelli [18]. The skin paddle is designed over the dorsoulnar aspect of the first metacarpal distal to the emergence of the dorsal branch of the radial artery in the first webspace. Dorsoulnar and dorsoradial arteries for the thumb branch out directly from the radial artery or from the first dorsal interosseous artery. This axial flap carries the

http://dx.doi.org/10.5772/intechopen.74152

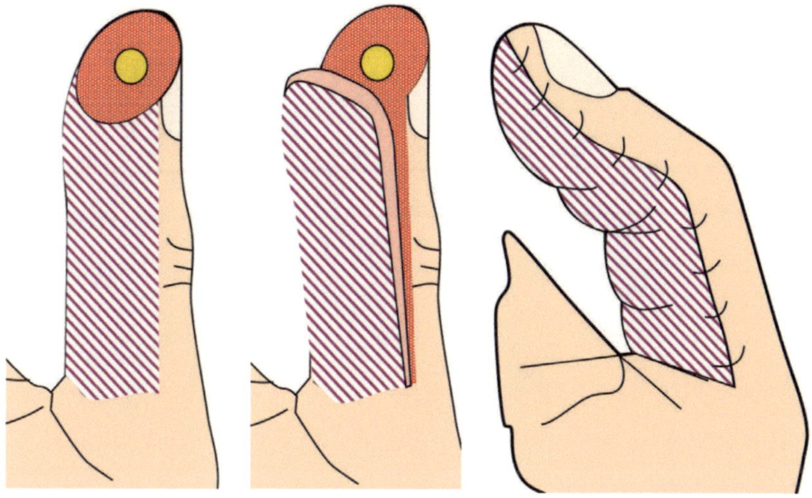

Figure 16. Möberg's flap.

dorsoulnar branch of the thumb which anastomoses with the thumb proper ulnar artery at the neck of the proximal phalanx. The dorsoulnar artery needs to be ligated proximal to the island paddle, and dissection is performed from distal to proximal (**Figures 17** and **18**).

The flap can potentially include radial sensory branches found near the dorsoulnar branch which can then be sutured to the proper digital nerve to attempt a sensate type of flap. Otherwise, this flap will not provide sensation to the tip of the thumb.

A similar flap has been described based on the dorsoradial artery of the thumb [19]. However, the dorsoulnar branch is considered more dominant and constant.

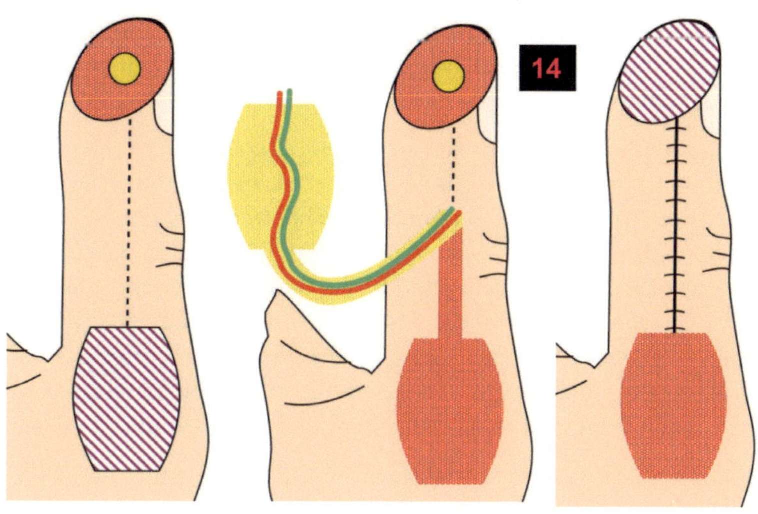

Figure 17. Brunelli's flap.

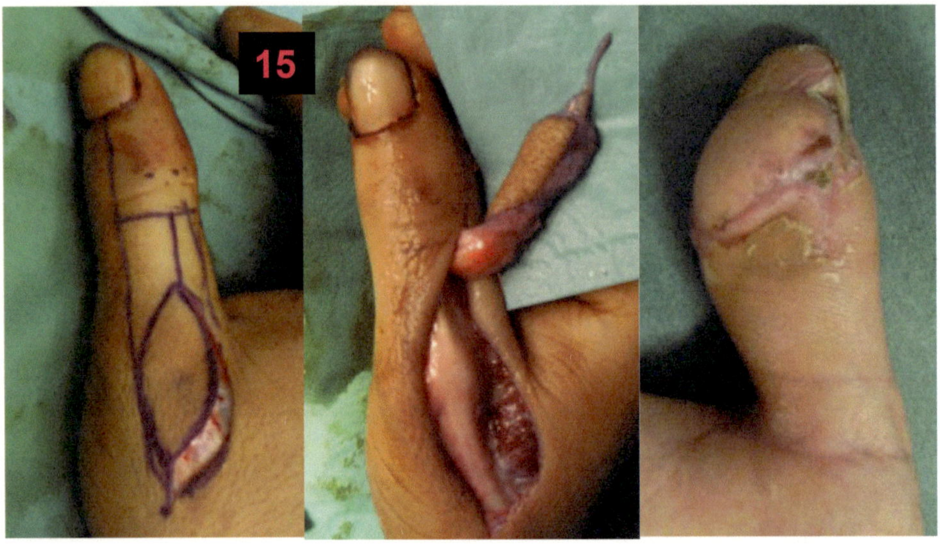

Figure 18. Clinical case of homodigital dorsoulnar retrograde flap for the tip of the thumb.

Cavadas [20] described a modification that included a small portion of the first metacarpal diaphysis. This was presented as an option for complex injuries with a severe bone defect at the distal phalanx.

6.6. Heterodigital flaps

6.6.1. Littler neurovascular island flap

Currently, this type of reconstruction has lost popularity. The previously described anterograde homodigital flaps and microsurgical procedures such as toe to pulp transfer have limited its use. It is still interesting in case of a spare skin paddle and corresponding neurovascular pedicle of an otherwise nonsalvageable digit. This can then be used to reconstruct other injured digits but mainly for thumb reconstruction (**Figure 19**).

The selected donor site is the ulnar aspect of the middle and ring fingers. The skin paddle is marked; it extends from the volar midline until the dorsal midline. The pedicle dissection must be continued until the superficial palmar arch has been reached. A cuff of perivascular tissue needs to be preserved; after releasing the natatory fibres of the palmar fascia, the proper digital artery of the adjacent finger is ligated at the bifurcation of the common palmar digital artery, and the dissection of the pedicle is then accomplished up to the superficial arch. Brunner and hemi-Brunner types of incisions in both zone II and zone III have to be done in order to reach the proper pedicle length. The island flap has to be transferred without tension, kinking or compression through a subcutaneous tunnel to the thumb.

The sensory integration of the flap is variable, and the older the patient is, the less recognition will take place. However, this is not essential to reach adequate function.

The donor site needs skin grafting.

http://dx.doi.org/10.5772/intechopen.74152

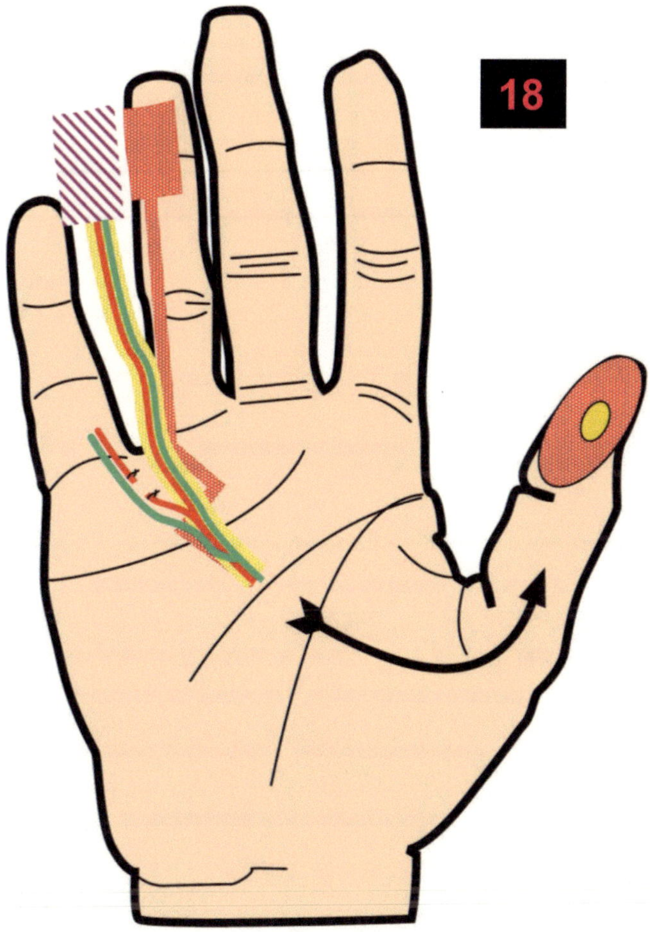

Figure 19. Littler's flap and heterodigital hemipulp neurovascular flap.

6.7. Metacarpal artery island flaps

6.7.1. First dorsal metacarpal artery flap

The so-called cerf-volant was described by Foucher and Braun [21] and has been considered the main workhorse in thumb reconstruction (**Figures 20** and **21**).

Based on the first dorsal metacarpal artery (FDMA), which is a branch of the dorsal radial artery of the hand, it courses parallel to the first metacarpal bone and superficial to the first dorsal interosseous muscle fascia although some fibres may cover the vessel at its course. The FDMA has vascular connections with the PDA at the level of the metacarpal neck.

The island paddle is outlined at the dorsal skin of the proximal phalanx. It extends from the PIP joint to the MCP joint. Laterally, it can extend from the radial midline to the ulnar midline of the finger. Dissection has to be carried out subfascially in order not to damage the pedicle.

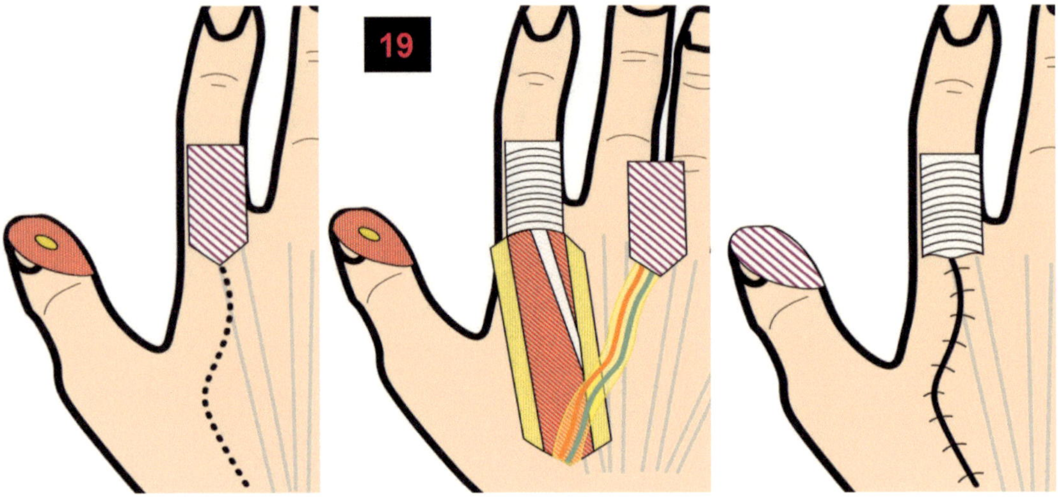

Figure 20. Cerf-volant Foucher's flap, based on the first dorsal interosseous artery.

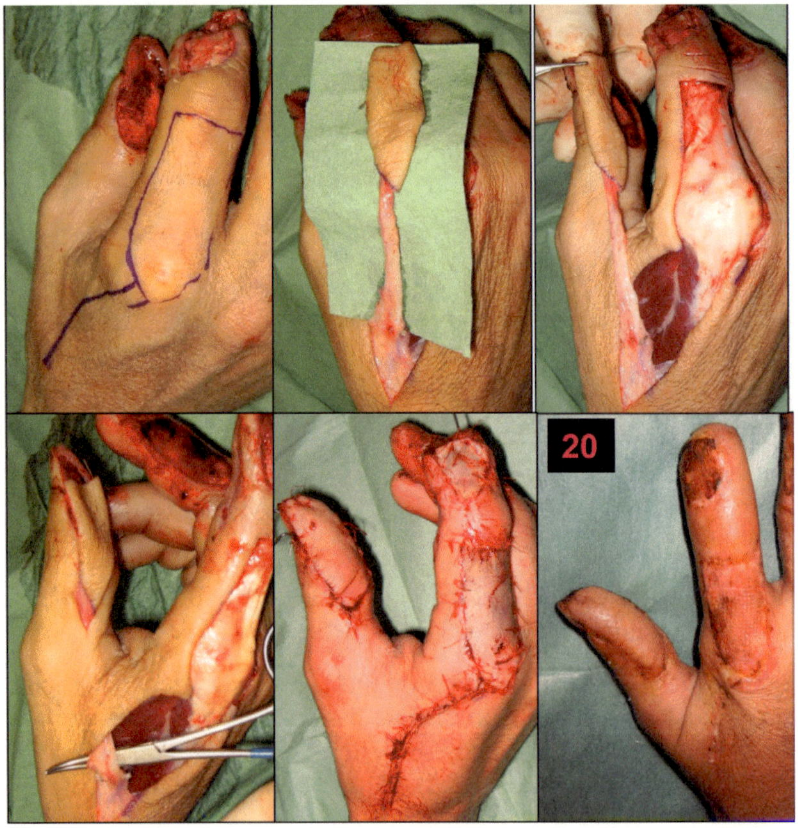

Figure 21. Clinical case of a defect of the tip of the thumb treated with a Foucher's flap.

http://dx.doi.org/10.5772/intechopen.74152

A lazy S incision is performed from the MCP joint to the anatomic snuffbox. The pedicle is then released until its emergency at the dorsal radial artery. Subcutaneous veins and sensory branches of the radial nerve are identified and can be included in the flap.

A tunnel is dissected from the first interosseous webspace to the defect at the tip of the thumb, and the flap and its pedicle are transferred and sutured. The pedicle must not be compressed under the tunnel, and the flap should be sutured tension-free.

6.7.2. *Reverse-flow dorsal metacarpal flaps*

The dorsal metacarpal arteries (DMA) are branches of the dorsal arch supplied by the radial artery. They course underneath the extensor tendons, included in the epimysial lining of the dorsal interosseous muscles (**Figures 22** and **23**).

Due to the vascular connections with the deep palmar arch through recurrent cutaneous branches, this flap can be raised retrogradely. These connections are found distal to the juncturae tendinum.

Early and Milner [22] developed a reverse-flow island flap, based on the dorsal metacarpal arteries. This flap includes the whole course of the metacarpal artery; at the proximal end, the artery is ligated. The dissection must leave the peritenon of the extensor tendon intact

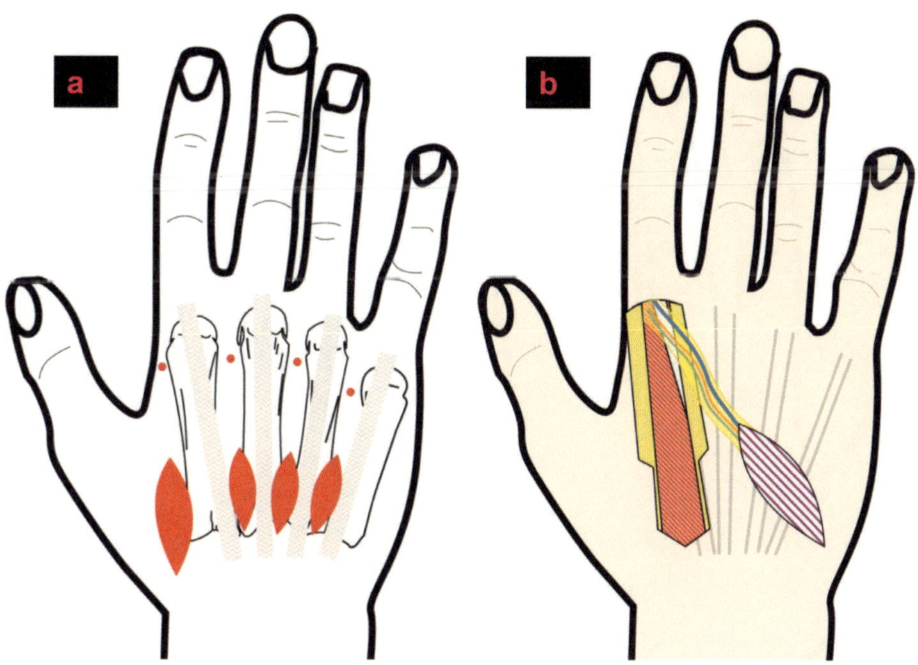

Figure 22. Dorsal metacarpal flaps of reverse flow: (a) position of the skin paddles (ellipses) and pivotal points (red dots); (b) the pedicle includes the fascia of the dorsal interosseous muscle.

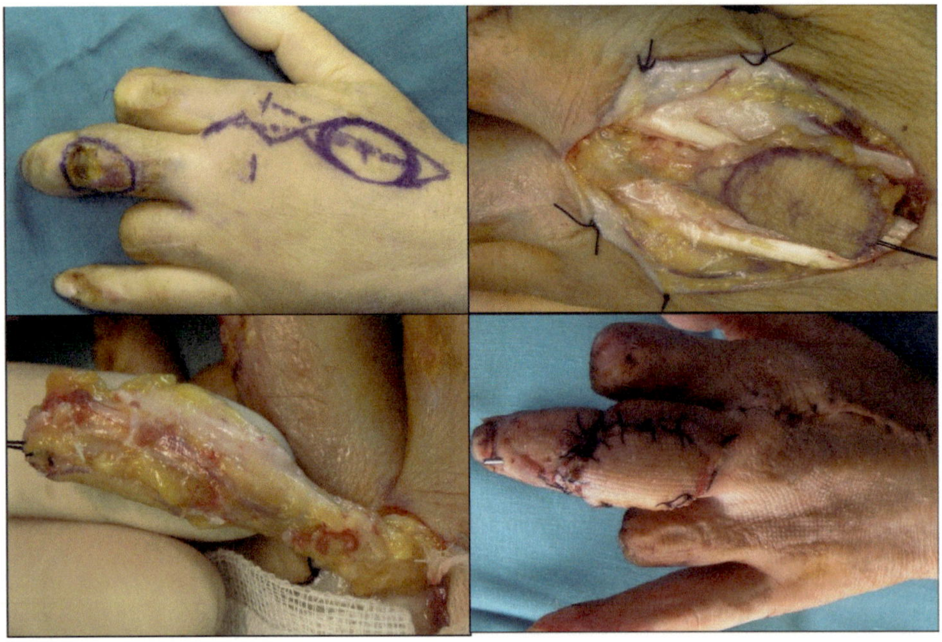

Figure 23. Clinical case of skin defect on the proximal interphalangeal joint of the middle finger; the second dorsal metacarpal artery flap is performed.

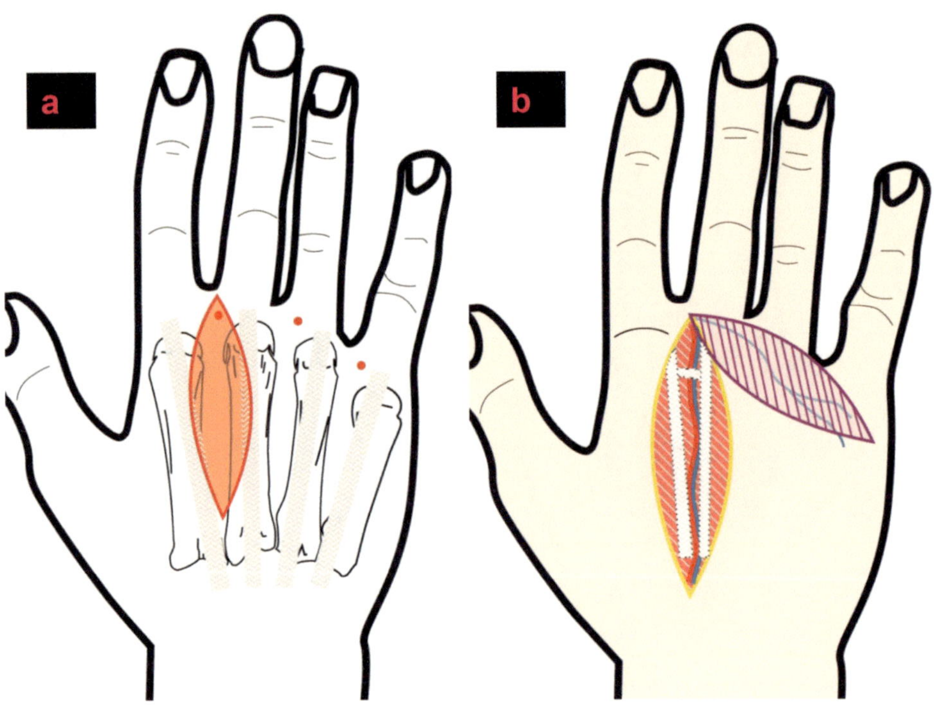

Figure 24. Quaba Davison's flaps: (a) location of the skin paddles (ellipses) and pivotal points (red dots); (b) the flap does not include the fascia of the dorsal interosseous muscle, and the pivotal point is immediately distal to the juncturae tendinum.

http://dx.doi.org/10.5772/intechopen.74152

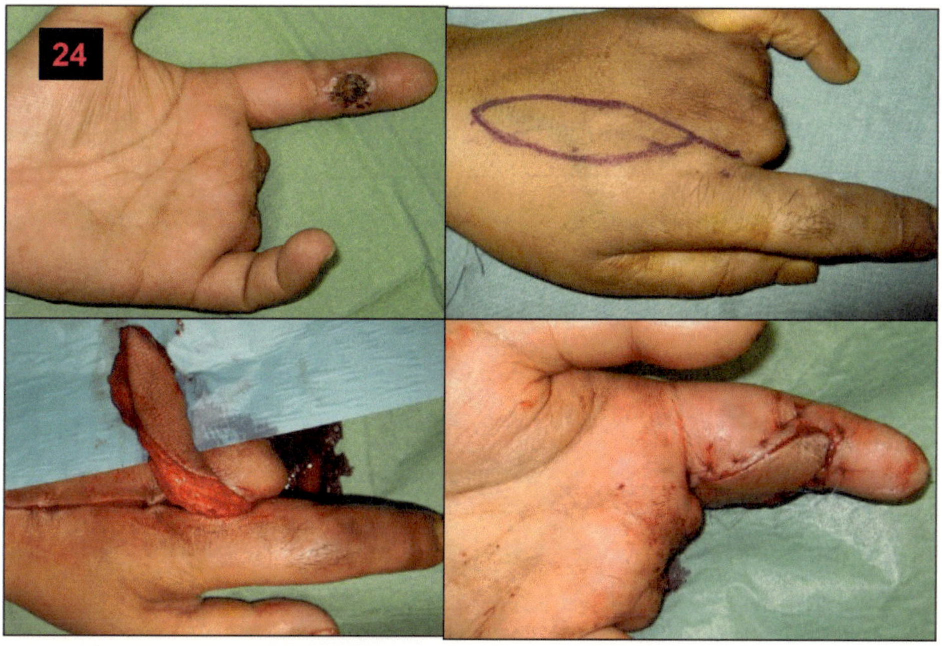

Figure 25. Clinical case of a volar defect at the medial phalanx: a Quaba Davison's flap was used since many of the adjacent digits had been amputated.

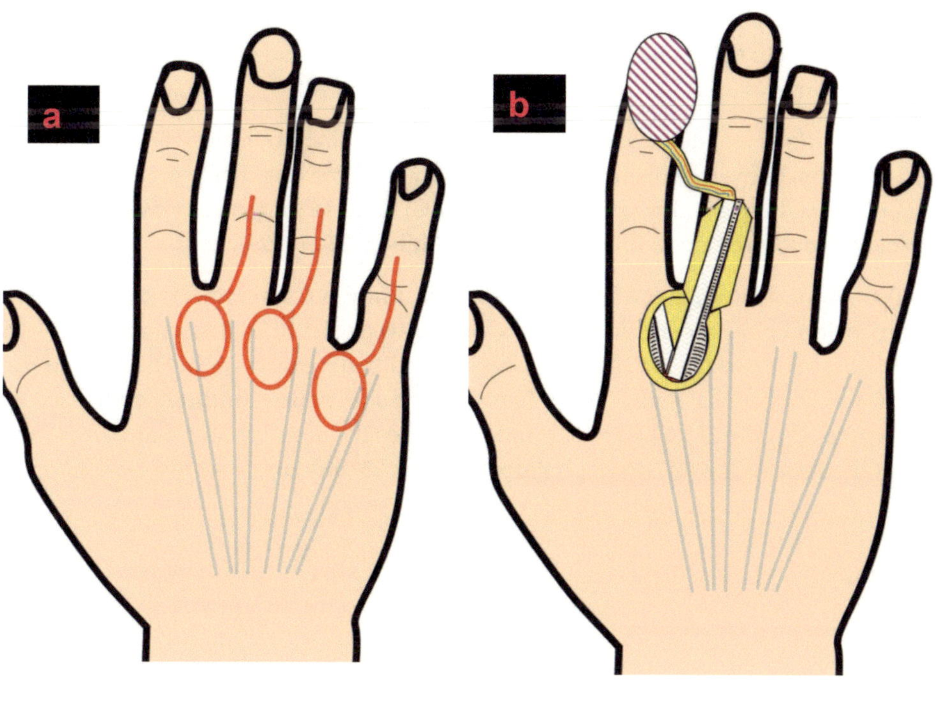

Figure 26. Dorsal commissural flaps: (a) location of the skin paddles (ellipses); (b) the flap reaches the distal interphalangeal joints and the distal phalanx.

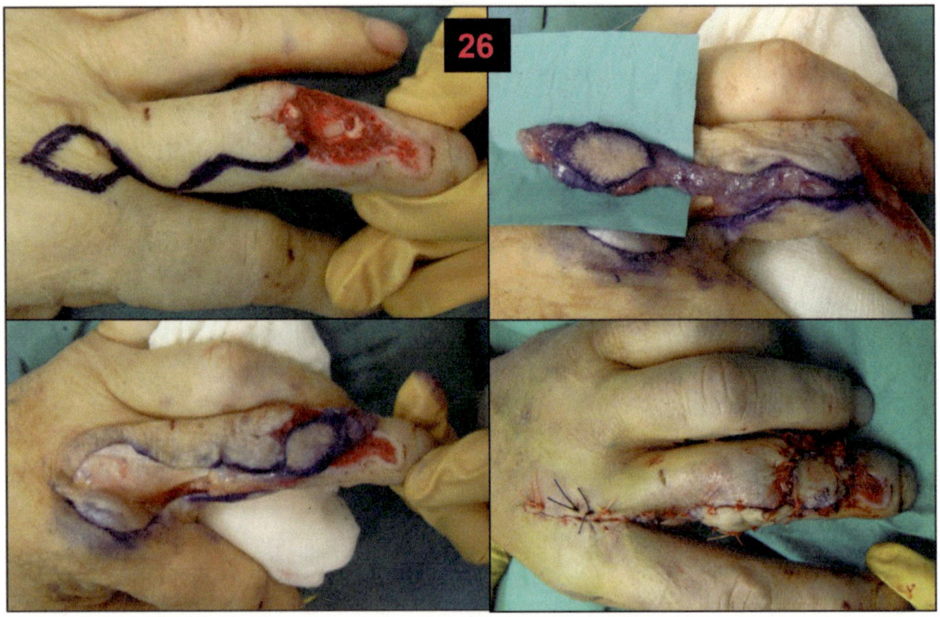

Figure 27. Clinical case of soft tissue defect on the medial phalanx where a dorsal commissural flap was obtained.

and include the interosseous fascia. The juncturae must be released, and dissection has to end at the level of the metacarpal neck. Dorsal sensory branches and possible veins must be included in the flap. The island paddle extends from the MCP joint to the wrist crease. The arc of rotation of this flap (180°) allows the coverage of the proximal phalanx and PIP joint up to the middle phalanx.

Quaba and Davidson [23] described the same flap without incorporating the DMA (**Figures 23** and **24**). Dissection of the flap proceeds suprafascially, and it is based only on the recurrent cutaneous branch. The flap can also extend from the MCP joint to the wrist crease. The flap is then easier to elevate and provides a thinner coverage (**Figures 25** and **26**).

Eventually, anatomic studies confirmed the existence of vascular connections at different levels of the proximal phalanx and medial phalanx between the PDA and cutaneous braches of the DMA. Karacalar and Özcan [24] described a modified version of this flap based on these anatomic findings. This is a reverse-flow flap with the skin paddle outlined on the second and third webspaces (**Figure 27**). The arc of rotation reaches the distal phalanx, and the pivot point is found at the neck of the proximal phalanx (**Figures 25** and **26**).

7. Summary

Local hand flaps offer excellent coverage of soft tissue loss when a skin graft is not eligible and when the defect is small or moderate.

http://dx.doi.org/10.5772/intechopen.74152

The knowledge of the neurovascular anatomy is paramount in order to understand and perform these flaps.

Most local flaps provide adequate sensation and cosmesis using locoregional skin. However, local flaps obviously have limited indications, and larger or complex cases need a microsurgical approach instead of or even further amputation if considered nonsalvageable. Surgeons should recognize which indication is correct in every case.

Author details

Francisco Martinez Martinez[1]*, M. Llanos Guerrero Navarro[2], Juan Garcia Navarro[1], Alberto Gimenez Ros[1] and Alba Izquierdo Robledano[1]

*Address all correspondence to: fmtnez@gmail.com

1 Hospital Universitario Virgen de la Arrixaca, Murcia, Spain

2 Hospital General Universitario Santa Lucia, Cartagena, Murcia, Spain

References

[1] Littler JW. Neurovascular pedicle transfer of tissue in reconstructive surgery of the hand. The Journal of Bone and Joint Surgery. American Volume. 1956;**38**:917

[2] Lister GD, Gibson T. Closure of rhomboid skin defects: The flaps of Limberg and Dufourmentel. British Journal of Plastic Surgery. 1972;**25**(3):300-314

[3] Foucher G, Braun JB. A new island flap transfer from the dorsum of the index to the thumb. Plastic and Reconstructive Surgery. 1979;**63**(3):344-349

[4] Yang G, Chen B, Gao Y. The forearm free skin flap transplantation. National Medical Journal of China. 1981;**61**:139

[5] Medalie DA. Perforator-based forearm and hand adipofascial flaps for the coverage of difficult dorsal hand wounds. Annals of Plastic Surgery. 2002;**48**(5):477-483

[6] Orbay JL, Rosen JG, Khouri RK, et al. The glabrous palmar flap: The new free or reversed pedicled palmar fasciocutaneous flap for volar hand reconstruction. Techniques in Hand & Upper Extremity Surgery. 2009;**13**(3):145-150

[7] Zancolli EA, Angrigiani C. Posterior interosseous island forearm flap. Journal of Hand Surgery British. 1988;**13**(2):130-135

[8] Bertelli JA, Pagliei A. The neurocutaneous flap based on the dorsal branches of the ulnar artery and nerve. A new flap for extensive reconstruction of the hand. Plastic and Reconstructive Surgery. 1998;**101**(6):1537-1543

[9] Cronin TD. The cross finger flap: A new method of repair. The American Surgeon. 1951; **17**(5):419-425

[10] Tranquilli-Leali E. Reconstruzione del apice falangi vaguali mediante autoplástica volare pedunculata per scorimento. Infort Traum Lavoro. 1935;**1**:186-193

[11] Atasoy E, Ioakimidis E, Kasdan ML, et al. Reconstruction of the amputated finger tip with a triangular volar flap. Journal of Bone and Joint Surgery. 1970;**52**:921-926

[12] Kutler W. A new method for fingertip amputation. Journal of the American Medical Association. 1947;**133**(1):29-30

[13] Venkataswami DR, Subramanian N. Oblique triangular flap: A new method of repair for oblique amputations of the fingertip and thumb. Plastic and Reconstructive Surgery. 1980;**66**(2):296-300

[14] Hueston JT. Local flap repair of fingertip injuries. Plastic and Reconstructive Surgery. 1966;**37**(4):349-350

[15] Lai CS, Ling SD, Yang CC. The reverse digital artery flap for fingertip reconstruction. Annals of Plastic Surgery. 1989;**22**(6):495-500

[16] Moberg E. Aspects of sensation in reconstructive surgery of the upper extremity. The Journal of Bone and Joint Surgery. American Volume. 1964;**46**:817-825

[17] O'Brien B. Neurovascular island pedicle flaps for terminal amputations and digital scars. British Journal of Plastic Surgery. 1968;**21**(3):258-261

[18] Brunelli F, Vigasio A, Valenti P, Brunelli GR. Arterial anatomy and clinical application of the dorsoulnar flap of the thumb. Journal of Hand Surgery. 1999;**24**(4):803-811

[19] Bakhach J, Sentucq-Rigal J, Mouton P, Boileau R, Panconi B, Guimberteau JC. The dorsoradial flap: A new flap for hand reconstruction. Anatomical study and clinical applications. Annales de Chirurgie Plastique et Esthétique. 2006;**51**(1):53-60

[20] Cavadas P. Reverse osteocutaneous dorsoulnar thumb flap. Plastic and Reconstructive Surgery. 2003;**111**(1):326-329

[21] Foucher G, Braun J. A new island flap transfer from the dorsum of the index to the thumb. Plastic and Reconstructive Surgery. 1979;**62**(3):344-349

[22] Early MJ, Milner RH. Dorsal metacarpal flaps. British Journal of Plastic Surgery. 1987; **10**:333-341

[23] Quaba AA, Davidson PM. The distally-based dorsal hand flap. British Journal of Plastic Surgery. 1990;**43**(1):28-39

[24] Karacalar A, Özcan M. A new approach to the reverse dorsal metacarpal artery flap. Journal of Hand Surgery American. 1997;**22**(2):307-310

Chapter 8

Omental Flap in Breast Reconstruction

Ashraf Khater, Adel Fathi and Hosam Ghazy

Additional information is available at the end of the chapter

http://dx.doi.org/10.5772/intechopen.70115

Abstract

Objectives: The use of omental flap for breast reconstruction was reported by the Romanian surgeon Kiricuta in 1963, since that time some surgeons tried to use the omentum either pedicled or free for breast reconstruction. It can be used after partial or total mastectomy.

Aims: The aim of this chapter is to address indications, limitations, contraindications, and technique of omental flap for breast reconstruction.

Technique: This flap could be retrieved by either a small midline laparotomy or preferably by laparoscopic harvesting. Details of retrieval, tips and tricks are highlighted in this chapter.

Conclusions: Omental flap is a strong working horse in breast reconstruction after partial or skin sparing mastectomy (SSM). It can be free or pedicled. It could be retrieved by minilaparotomy or preferably by laparoscopic harvesting omental flap (LHOF). It is a simple, safe, and reliable flap that mimics the natural contour of the breast. In about 30% with volume insufficiency it can be used with an implant as a cover with low complication rate and good esthetic outcome.

Keywords: breast, reconstruction, omental flap, mastectomy

1. Historical background

The omentum is not just an abdominal structure, it is an unique organ with a peculiar location, shape, attachments, supply, and function. The omentum has a mechanical function as a barrier or sealant. It has an immune function and an endocrinal function through secreting many cytokines, growth factors, and hormones [1, 2]. Surgeons aimed to use this organ in many reconstructive procedures. The first use of a pedicled omental flap was reported by Senn in

1888 when he used it for protection of intestinal anastomosis [3]. More recently, the omentum was revisited by Knazozovicky in 1929 when he used the pedicled omentum after arthroplasty [4]. Due to its immune function, it was used for coverage of deep sternal and infected wounds as well as to protect anastomoses [5, 6]. The Romanian surgeon, Kiricuta described the use of the pedicled omental flap for repair of vesicovaginal fistula and for breast reconstruction after mastectomy [7, 8]. He reported on 10 cases of breast reconstruction after subcutaneous mastectomy with 40% pure omental reconstruction without any need for implants. This opened the gate for use of pedicled omental flap in breast reconstruction. The main two problems with this flap were the unpredictable volume [9, 10] and the requirement of laparotomy for retrieval. The latter was associated with potential morbidity especially in regards to the occurrence of incisional hernia [11]. Some researchers tried to extract this flap through a minilaparotomy; yet incisional hernia still remained a complication [12]. For this reason Saltz described omental flap retrieval through a laparoscopic approach [13]. Later on, there was a shift toward the laparoscopic retrieval with great success. The largest series was reported by Hisamitsu Zaha who performed around 200 cases of laparoscopically harvested omental flap (LHOF) with minimal complications and satisfactory aesthetic results [14]. Subsequently, to avoid any traction over the pedicle with added length of the pedicle to the total flap volume, a trend emerged toward usage of free omental flaps extracted through a small abdominal incision to avoid any traction over the pedicle with added length of the pedicle to the total flap volume [15, 16]. The first free omental flap was performed in an emergent basis to cover a large defect in the scalp after avulsion [15]. After that, its indications were widened and it was applied to several locations [17]. In this work, we shall try to answer the following question: is there a role for omental flap in breast reconstruction in the era of oncoplastic surgery?

2. Advantages of the omental flap

We can list several advantages of the omental flap [11, 12, 18]:

1. Easy harvest which is not technically demanding, and that is characterized by a short learning curve.
2. Minimal donor site morbidity especially with the use of laparoscopic harvesting.
3. Minimal blood loss.
4. Can be retrieved simultaneously with mastectomy by two teams with neither need for extra time nor for changing patient's position for staged operations.
5. Fast recovery with early discharge especially with laparoscopic harvesting.
6. This flap is fatty in nature, so it mimics the normal breast and you can hardly differentiate in between even with the use of mammography (**Figure 1**).
7. Reliability of its axial blood supply with less common ischemic complications transverse rectus abdominis myocutaneous flap (TRAM) is a perforator flap with common ischemic complications and fat necrosis.

8. Great adaptability to any cavities.

9. Great malleability with ease in reshaping to mimic the breast mound.

10. It is a good reconstructive tool in obese women (its volume increases with weight gain) and can be retrieved with the laparoscope without major complications. On the other hand, obesity is a relative contraindication for TRAM flap and its ischemic complications increases in obese women.

11. Long pedicle which can be transferred easily to the mastectomy bed through an epigastric incision.

12. The flap is bipedicled and can be divided to work for both breasts simultaneously.

13. It has a characteristic absorptive power, so seroma is less evident and drain output is usually of lesser amount.

14. It is the only flap that shows a unique phenomenon of size gain, which is completed by the end of the sixth month. Other flaps (or lipofilling) usually undergo size decrease with progress of time due to either muscle atrophy or adipose tissue loss [19].

15. It has an immune function and good tissue adherence, so it can cover ischemic areas.

16. It is suitable for all ages, stages, body weights, and controllable comorbidities.

17. It has a very good tolerance for postoperative radiotherapy.

18. Surprisingly, if it is used as a cover for the silicone implants, capsular contracture, and rupture are rare [12].

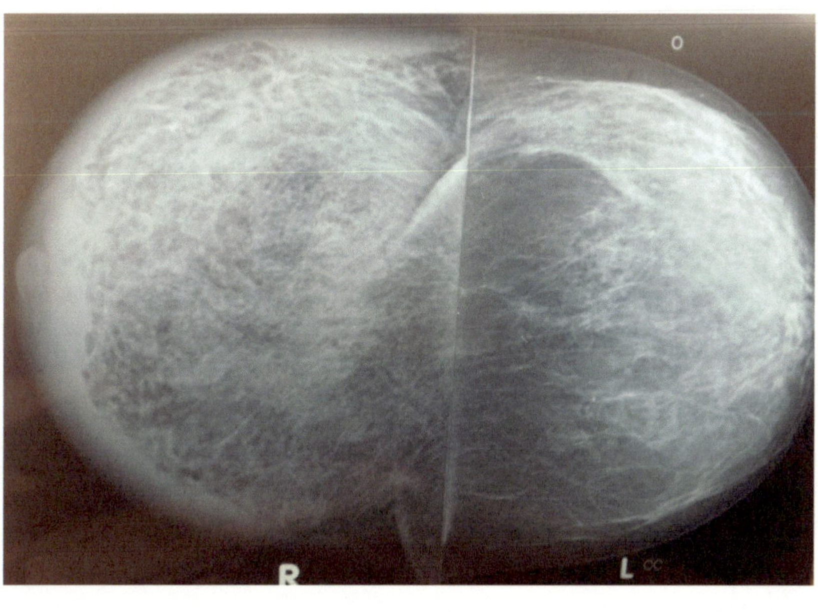

Figure 1. Mammographic view of the right breast reconstructed with an omental flap.

3. Limitations

1. The main drawback of this flap is the unpredictable volume, however if volume is insufficient [9, 11], it can be used safely as a cover for an implant.
2. It is not suitable for cases in which the whole breast with its skin is removed.
3. It may be deficient in thin women (implant can be used as an adjunct).
4. It is considered an abdominal operation with all hazards of laparoscopic use as bleeding, visceral injuries, and complications of laparoscopy.
5. Presence of adhesions may be a limiting factor.
6. Presence of peritoneal metastases or omental deposits may preclude flap retrieval.

3.1. Contraindications

1. The main contraindication is the presence of omental malignant nodules, omental cake, or malignant ascites [11].
2. If omentectomy was done for any reason.
3. Presence of marked abdominal adhesions that make retrieval difficult.
4. Contraindications of laparoscopy.

4. Anatomic considerations

The greater omentum is attached inferiorly to the transverse colon after making a loop over itself forming a four layer loop. Superiorly, it is attached to the greater curve of the stomach (**Figure 2**) [20–22].

It has the advantage of having a dual blood supply from both gastroepiploic arteries (right epiploic from gastroduodenal and left from the splenic). Both form anterior and posterior epiploic arcades (**Figure 3**) and gives rise to anterior, posterior, and accessory epiploic arteries.

The flap pedicle can be based on either the right or the left gastroepiploic arteries (commonly the right) after dividing the contralateral artery (**Figure 4**). However, if a free flap is used, both vascular pedicles can be anastomosed to the branches of the axillary artery through a microvascular anastomosis.

Moreover, the flap can be lengthened by dividing the anterior epiploic arteries keeping the anterior and posterior omental arcades (**Figure 5**).

http://dx.doi.org/10.5772/intechopen.70115

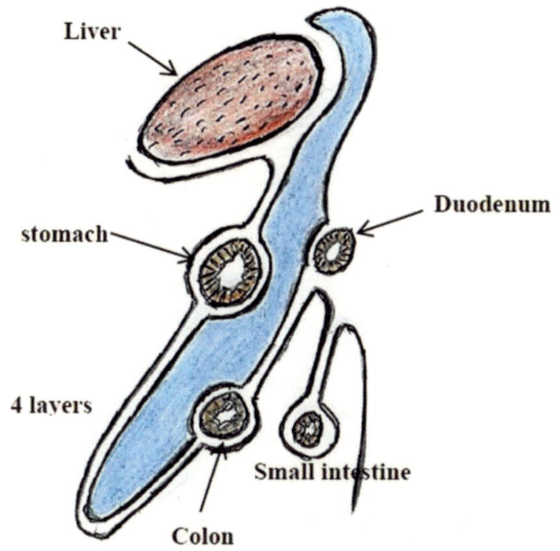

Figure 2. Layers and attachment of the greater omentum.

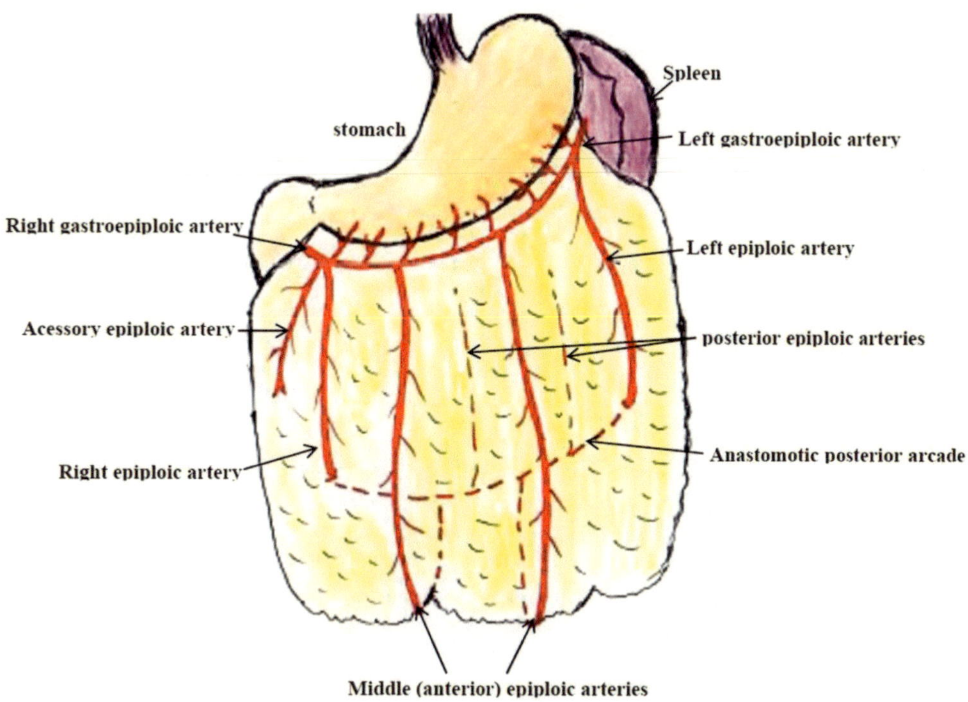

Figure 3. Arterial supply of the greater omentum.

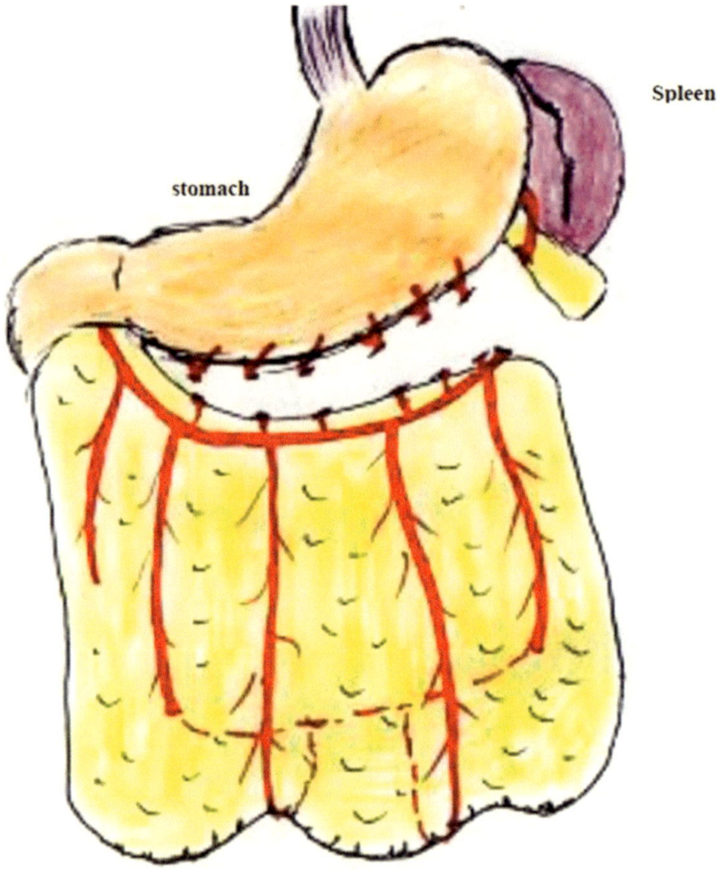

Figure 4. Pedicled omental flap based on the right gastroepiploic artery.

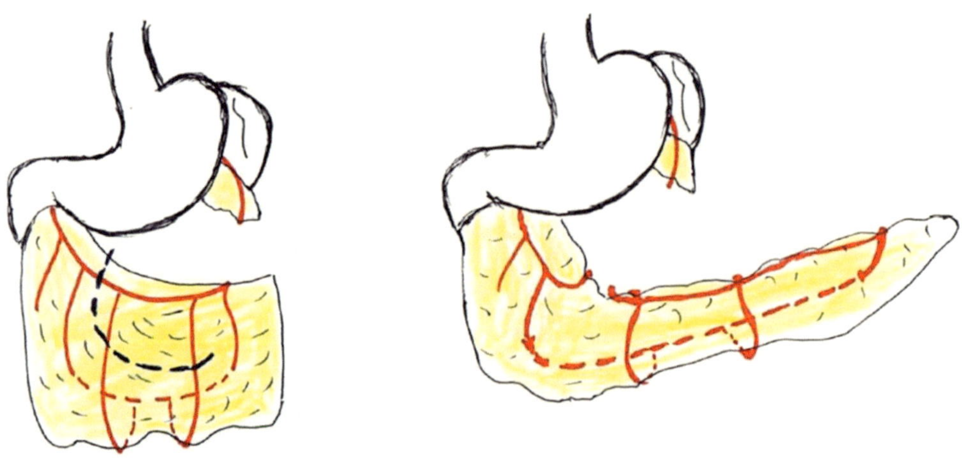

Figure 5. Lengthened omental flap (dotted division line).

http://dx.doi.org/10.5772/intechopen.70115

5. Technique

The omentum may be retrieved through a small epigastric minilaparotomy (**Figure 6**) or through laparoscopy. Laparoscopic ports are usually infra-umbilical; a 12 mm port just below the umbilicus for the camera and two 5 mm lateral ports for handling and dissection. Optional one or two 5 mm ports may be used in the upper right or left hypochondrium for omental retraction if it has a large volume (**Figure 7**).

In laparoscopic harvest, it is preferable to start dissection with separation of the omentum from the colonic attachment to preserve the flap suspended from the greater curve (**Figure 8**).

Then working in a counterclockwise direction, dissection is extended toward the left gastroepiploic artery which is sealed and divided either by harmonic scalpel or preferably by Ligasure as this device can control sizable vessels (**Figure 9**).

Then, we start dividing the attachment to the greater curvature of the stomach up to the visualization of the right gastroepiploic artery within a fold (**Figure 10**).

The last step is a creation of an epigastric incision through the lower mastectomy flap, then a 12 mm trocar is introduced to grasp the distal tip of the freed omentum which is widened to 2–3 fingers width to allow transmission of the flap to the mastectomy bed (**Figure 11**).

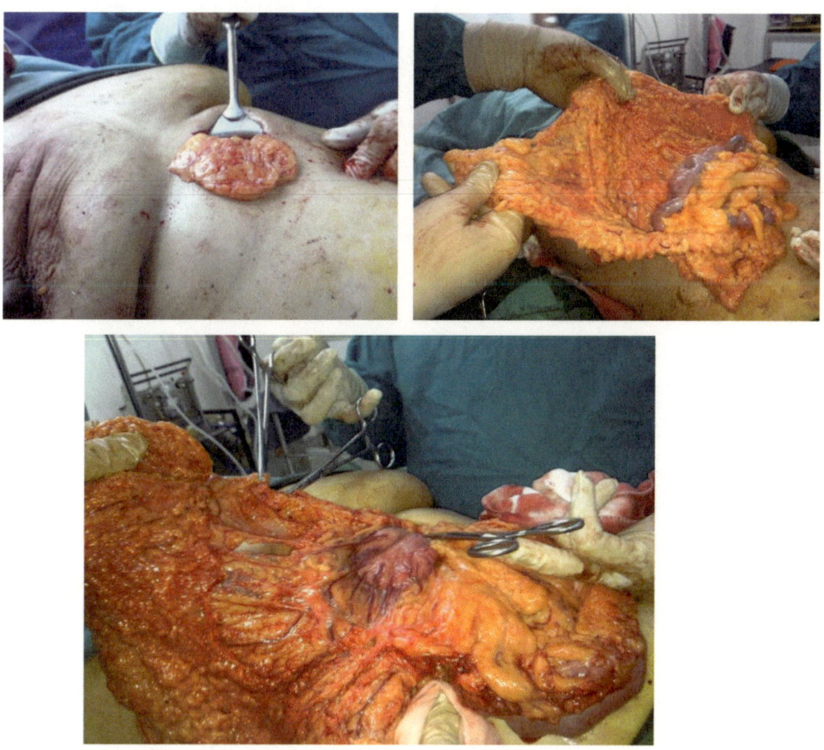

Figure 6. Omental flap retrieved through a small epigastric minilaparotomy.

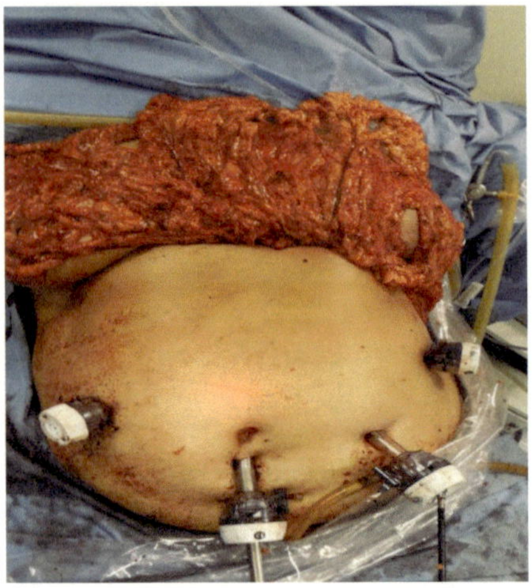

Figure 7. Laparoscopically retrieved omental flap with port sites demonstrated.

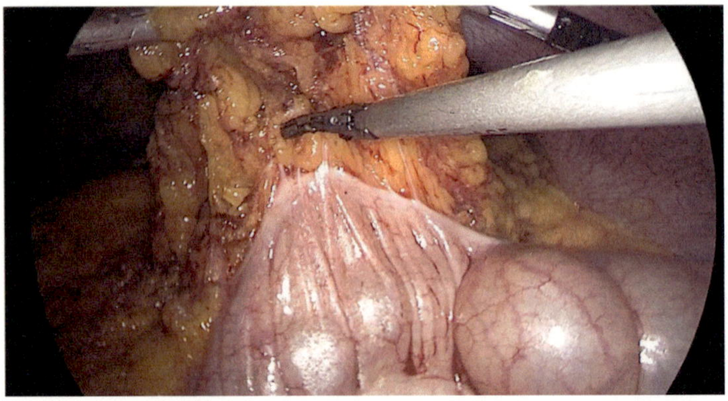

Figure 8. Separation of the greater omentum from the colonic attachment.

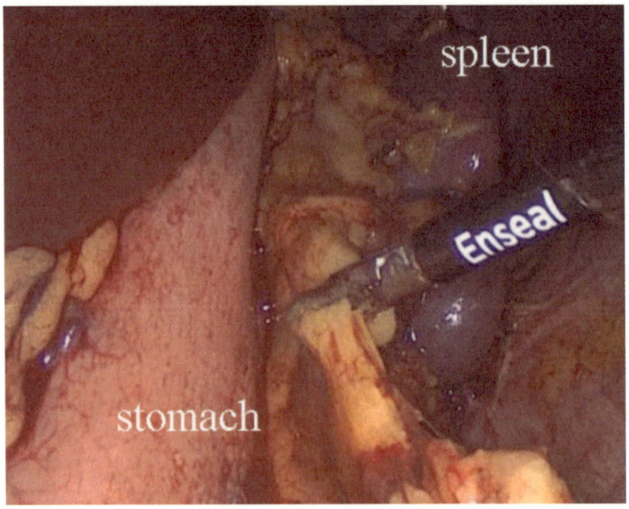

Figure 9. Division of the left gastroepiploic artery.

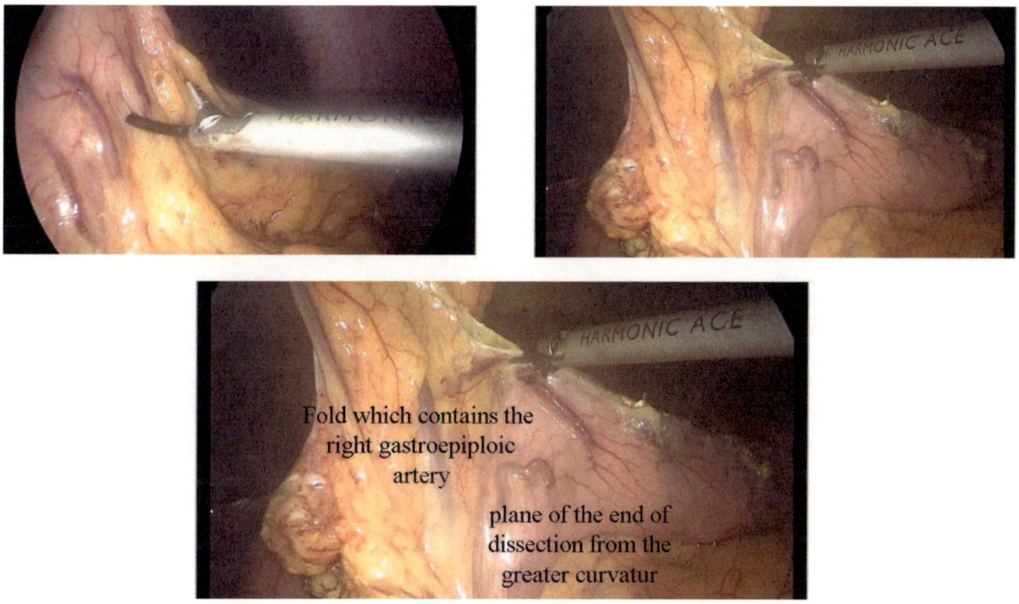

Figure 10. Division of attachments to the greater curvature.

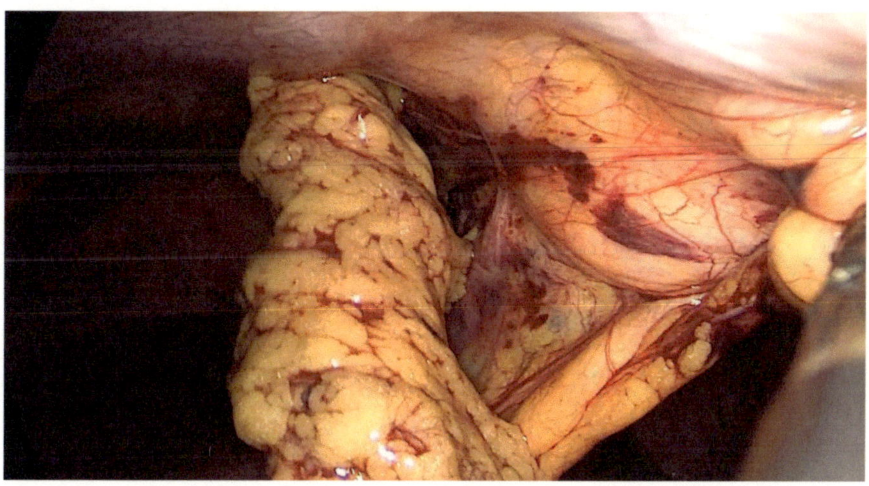

Figure 11. Grasping of the flap distal end to be transmitted into the mastectomy bed.

When the flap is transferred to the bed, it could be molded to fit to the breast envelope, then the flap should be fixed by few nonabsorbable sutures to the underlying muscles to avoid flap retraction into the abdomen. Care should be exercised to avoid injury of the vascular pedicle by these sutures. We prefer carrying mastectomy through a hidden inframammary incision close to the epigastrium. This allows delivery of the flap through the subcutaneous tunnel and enables us to obtain a very good cosmetic outcome "scarless procedure" (**Figure 12**). The problem with this incision is the relative higher ischemic complications, these can be avoided

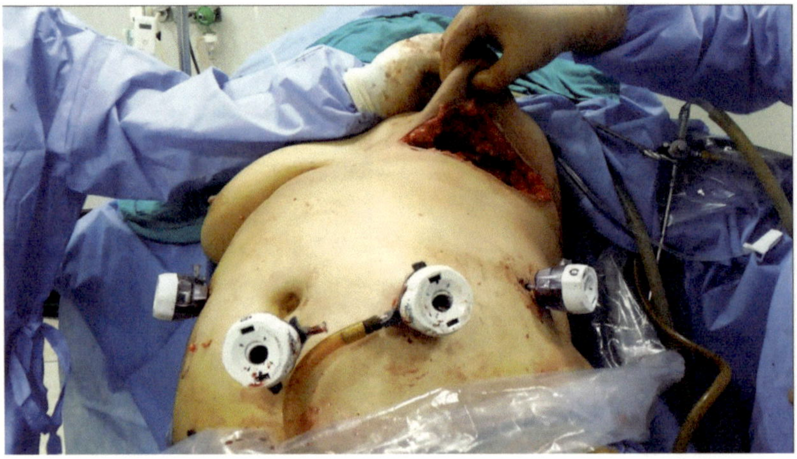

Figure 12. Inframammary incision to make a scarless procedure and to ease flap retrieval through the epigastric incision.

by testing its vascularity by either simple pricking, peripheral cutting or through dye techniques. However, any ischemia could be easily managed in the outpatient clinic with a very satisfactory cosmetic outcome.

6. Volume insufficiency

In the largest reported series by the Japanese surgeon Hisamitsu Zaha that included 200 cases, volume insufficiency was around 30%; in such case, a silicone implant could be used as an adjunct with a very good aesthetic outcome (**Figure 13**) [14].

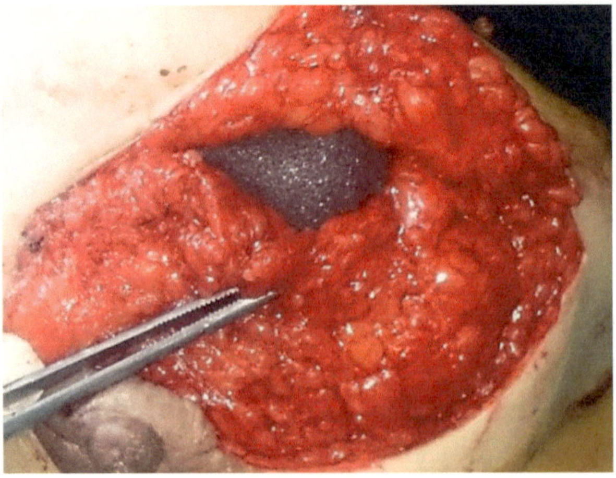

Figure 13. Silicone implant as an adjunct with omental flap.

http://dx.doi.org/10.5772/intechopen.70115

7. Pedicled versus free flaps

A free omental flap is recommended if remote coverage is required such as scalp avulsion, however there are advantages for free omental flap transfer in breast reconstruction, such as making benefit of the length of pedicle when added to the flap [16], ridding the patient of epigastric discomfort or pain due to passage of the pedicle through the tunnel, and finally minimal incidence of epigastric hernia consequent upon avoidance of the epigastric wound. This is especially so, if the omental flap is retrieved through a small Pfannenstiel incision or even through an epigastric wound which is completely closed.

8. Evaluation of flap integrity

Some authors leave a small window for this purpose, however the best way is to perform an intraoperative Doppler study and postoperative Duplex assessment (**Figure 14**).

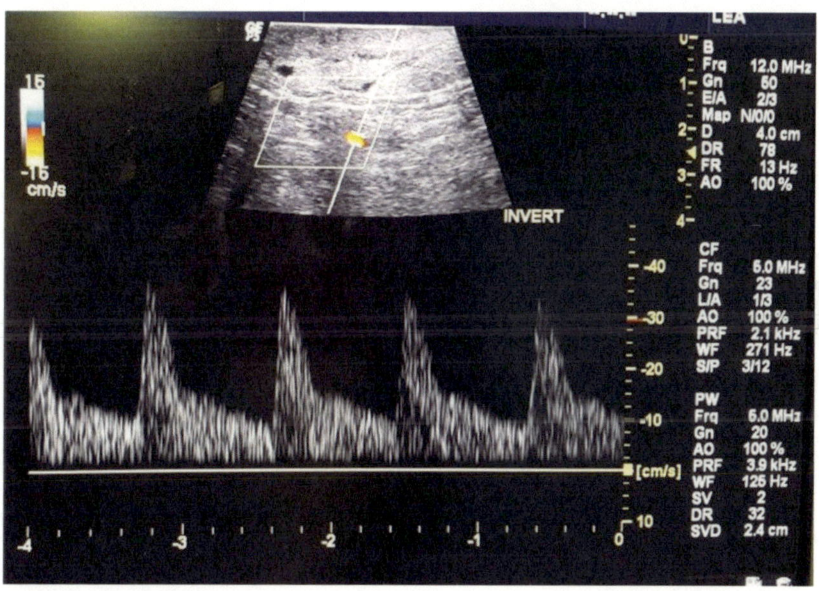

Figure 14. Duplex assessment showing an intact vascularity.

9. The aesthetic outcome

As reported by many authors, more than 80% of patients express an excellent aesthetic outcome [14]. **Figures 15** and **16** show cases of skin sparing mastectomy (SSM) reconstructed with a pedicled omental flap. In **Figure 15**, retrieval was done through a minlaparotomy and in **Figure 16** it was through a laparoscopic harvesting (LHOF) with a nearly scarless procedure.

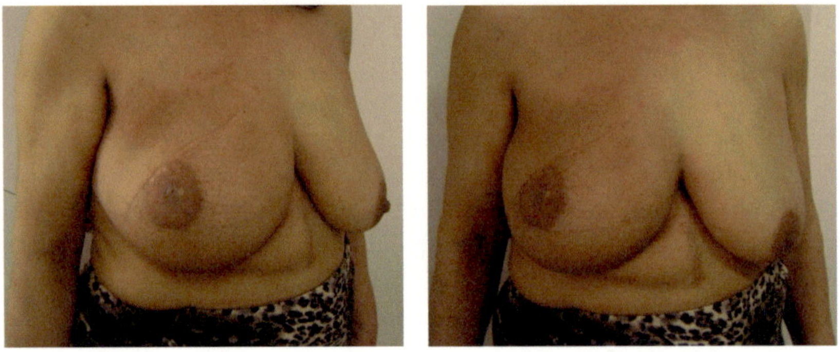

Figure 15. SSM which is reconstructed with pedicled omental flap through minilaparotomy.

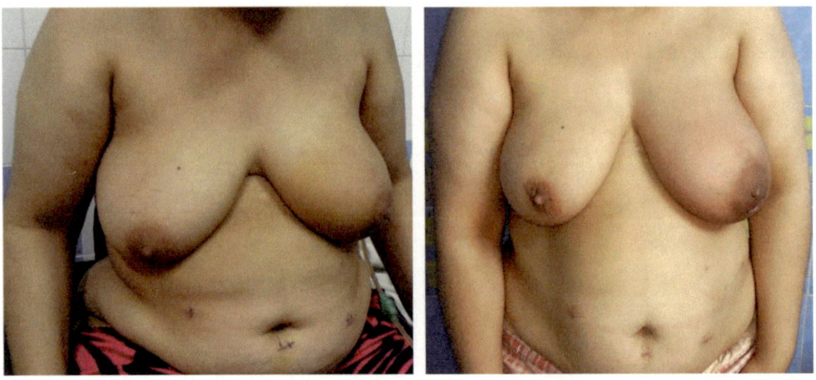

Figure 16. SSM which is reconstructed with laparoscopically harvested omental flap (LHOF).

10. Complications

10.1. General

1. Those of laparoscopy, as complications of the access, visceral injury, gas embolism, etc.
2. Chest complications.
3. Deep venous thrombosis (DVT) and pulmonary embolism.

10.2. Specific

1. Flap loss which may be either total or partial (partial loss may be minor or major that mandates surgical resection).
2. Traumatic fat necrosis.

http://dx.doi.org/10.5772/intechopen.70115

3. Local sepsis that may end up with necrotizing fasciitis especially in poorly controlled diabetics; this may be another cause of flap loss.

4. Hemorrhage, either in the mastectomy bed or intra-abdominal after flap retrieval. The most common abdominal sources are, the sealed left gastroepiploic vessels, short gastric vessels, or sealed vessels along the greater curve.

5. Epigastric discomfort or hernia due to passage of the pedicle through the epigastric tunnel.

6. Port site hernia after laparoscopic retrieval.

7. Seroma which is less common than with mastectomy alone due to the absorptive power of this flap.

11. Place of the omental flap in the era of oncoplastic surgery

This flap is ideal to solve the problem of volume replacement of medial quadrant volume replacement in cases of partial mastectomy for tumors in the medial quadrant. Moreover, it is a very good choice for total breast reconstruction after skin sparing mastectomy (SSM) especially in women with body mass index above the age of 30 years. This is particularly so, even if the volume is not adequate, because in such case it can be used to cover a silicone implant to avoid the capsular contracture and implant rupture.

12. Conclusion

Omental flap is a strong working horse in breast reconstruction after partial or skin sparing mastectomy. It can be free or pedicled. It could be retrieved by a minilaparotomy or preferably by laparoscopic harvesting (LHOF). It is a simple, safe, and reliable flap that mimics the natural contour of the breast. In about 30% of cases with volume insufficiency, it can be used with an implant as a cover with low complication rate and good aesthetic outcome.

Author details

Ashraf Khater[1]*, Adel Fathi[1] and Hosam Ghazy[2]

*Address all correspondence to: dr.ashrafkhater@yahoo.com

1 Department of Surgical Oncology, Faculty of Medicine, Mansoura Oncology Center (OCMU), Mansoura University, Egypt

2 General Surgery Department, Mansoura University Hospital, Mansoura University, Egypt

References

[1] Smitka K, Marešová D. Adipose tissue as an endocrine organ: An update on pro-inflammatory and anti-inflammatory microenvironment. Prague Medical Report. 2015;**116**:(2):87-111

[2] Fonseca-Alaniz MH. Takada J. Alonso-Vale MI, Lima FB. The adipose tissue as a regulatory center of the metabolism. Arquivos Brasileiros de Endocrinologia & Metabologia. 2006;**50**:216-229

[3] Senn N. An experimental contribution to intestinal surgery, with special reference to the treatment of intestinal obstruction (concluded). Annals of Surgery. 1888;**7**:421-430

[4] Lieberman-Meffert D, White H. The Greater Omentum: Anatomy, Physiology, Pathology, Surgery, with a Historical Survey. New York: Springer; 1983

[5] Irons GB, Witzke DJ, Arnold PG, Wood MB. Use of the omental free flap for soft-tissue reconstruction. Annals of Plastic Surgery. 1983;**11**(6):501-507

[6] Parissis H, Al-Alao B, Soo A, Orr D, Young V. Risk analysis and outcome of mediastinal wound and deep mediastinal wound infections with specific emphasis to omental transposition. Journal of Cardiothoracic Surgery. Sep 2011;**6**:111

[7] Kiricuta I. The use of the great omentum in the surgery of breast cancer. La Presse Médicale. 1963;**5**:15-17

[8] Kiricuta I, Goldstein AM. The repair of extensive vesicovaginal fistulas with pedicled omentum: A review of 27 cases. The Journal of Urology. 1972;**108**:724-727

[9] Cothier-Savey I, Tamtawi B, Franck D, et al. Immediate breast reconstruction using laparoscopically harvested omental flap. Plastic and Reconstructive Surgery. 2001;**107**: 1156-1163

[10] Zaha H, Inamine S, Naito T, Nomura H. Laparoscopically harvested omental flap for immediate breast reconstruction. The American Journal of Surgery. Oct 2006;**192**(4):556-558

[11] Zaha H, Inamine S. Laparoscopically harvested omental flap: Results for 96 patients. Surgical Endoscopy. 2010;**24**:103-107

[12] Khater A. Erratum to: Evaluation of pedicled omental flap delivered through a minilaparotomy for immediate breast reconstruction in obese patients. Aesthetic Plastic Surgery. 2014;**38**:482

[13] Saltz R, Stowers R, Smith M, Gadacz TR. Laparoscopically harvested omental free flap to cover a large soft tissue defect. Annals of Surgery. 1993;**217**(5):542-546; discussion 6-7

[14] Zaha H, Abe N, Sagawa N, Unesoko M. Oncoplastic surgery with omental flap reconstruction: A study of 200 cases. Breast Cancer Research and Treatment. Jan 24, 2017;**162**(2):267-274. DOI: 10.1007/s10549-017-4124-9. [Epub ahead of print]

[15] McLean DH, Buncke HJ. Autotransplant of omentum to a large scalp defect, with microsurgical revascularization. Plastic and Reconstructive Surgery. 1972;**49**(3):268-274

[16] Gomez JA, Pascal SG, Michel S, Mitchel H, Richard L. Free omental flap for skin-sparing breast reconstruction harvested laparoscopically. Plastic & Reconstructive Surgery. 2002;**110**(2):545-551

[17] Losken A, Carlson GW, Culbertson JH, Scott Hultman C, Kumar AV, Jones GE, Bostwick 3rd J, Jurkiewicz MJ. Omental free flap reconstruction in complex head and neck deformities. Head & Neck. Apr 2002;**24**(4):326-331

[18] Costa SS, Blotta RM, Mariano MB, Meurer L, Edelweiss MIA. Laparoscopic treatment of Poland's syndrome using the omentum flap technique. Clinics Sao Paulo. 2010;**65**(4):401-406

[19] Costa SS, Blotta RM, Meurer L, Edelweiss MIA. Adipocyte morphometric evaluation and angiogenesis in the omentum transposed to the breast: A preliminary study. Clinics Sao Paulo. Feb 2011;**66**(2):307-312

[20] Skandalakis JE, Colborn GL, Weidman TA, Foster Jr RS, Kingsnorth AN, et al. Surgical Anatomy: The Embryologic and Anatomic Basis of Modern Surgery. Chapter 10. Peritoneum, Omenta, and Internal Hernias. Athens, Greece: Paschalidis Medical Publications; 2004

[21] Nakao K, Miyata M, Ito T, et al. Omental transposition and skin graft in patients for advanced or recurrent breast cancer. The Japanese Journal of Surgery. 1986;**16**:112

[22] Samson R, Pasternak BM. Current status of surgery of the omentum. Surgery, Gynecology & Obstetrics. 1979;**149**:437

Chapter 9

An Overview of Hypospadias Surgery

Wenceslao M. Calonge and Gianluca Sapino

Additional information is available at the end of the chapter

http://dx.doi.org/10.5772/intechopen.69924

Abstract

Performed by urologists and paediatric surgeons, hypospadias procedures go unnoticed in many classical treatises of plastic surgery. Hypospadias is a very common malformation that occurs in nearly 1 in 250 male births. It consists of an abnormal opening of the urethral meatus at some point of its dorsal aspect. It is associated with an incomplete, semi-circumferential foreskin and in nearly half of the patients it may be accompanied with a curvature of the penile shaft called chordee. Most classifications differentiate between distal, middle and proximal presentations. Different techniques have been proposed for its treatment; some of the most usual ones are briefly revised. Continued improvement in surgical management has made currently practised one-stage repairs possible. We provide an introduction to the current techniques, as well as operative tips and an overview of the most common pitfalls the surgeon must bear in mind when treating this condition.

Keywords: hypospadias, microsurgery, urethra, penoscrotal transposition, child, paediatrics, urology, congenital malformations

1. Introduction and classification

Derived from the Greek prefix *hypo* (under) and *spadon* (gap, cleft), the word hypospadias refers to a congenital condition in which the urethral meatus appears proximal to its usual location at the tip of the penis.

The urethral orifice may lie at any level on the *embryologic* dorsal[1] surface of penis, scrotum or even perineum. The foreskin lacks an inferior portion in a way that the remaining semi-circumferential

[1]Note that the embryological dorsal aspect of the urethra is named as *ventral* or *anterior* in many texts. This confusion probably derives from the surgeon's view of an exposed operative field on the table. A defect on the embryological ventral surface of the urethra corresponds to the condition known as epispadias.

tissue resembles of a hood. The glans itself may be slightly flattened. Moreover, many cases of hypospadias may present with a curvature named chordee (from Latin *chorda,* string) between glans and meatus. This chordee is usually produced by an excess of fibrous tissue.

In order to evaluate the location of the urethral meatus, it should be examined under mild retraction of the foreskin and the skin surrounding the orifice. Though there is no total consensus, most urological texts describe the level of the urethral meatus as follows (**Figure 1**):

- Distal or anterior (glandular and coronal)
- Middle (penile)
- Proximal or posterior (penoscrotal, scrotal and perineal).

All observations should include the degree of curvature. This is usually expressed by the angle between the main axis from basis and the main axis from the apex of the glans (**Figure 2**).

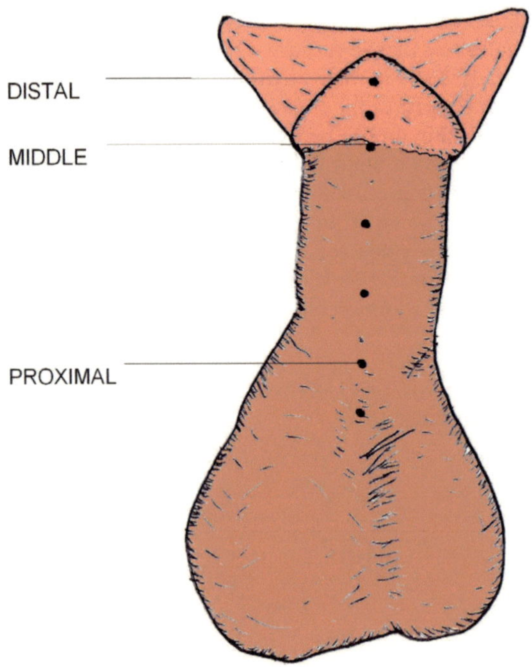

Figure 1. Classification of hypospadias according to level of the urethral meatus.

2. Historical notes

Most historical studies [1–3] refer to Heliodorus and Antyllus, two alexandrine surgeons who proposed total amputation of the penis distal to the orifice. The first description of hypospadias, however, is attributed to Galen (129-ca.199 AD). Several isolated observations and

http://dx.doi.org/10.5772/intechopen.69924

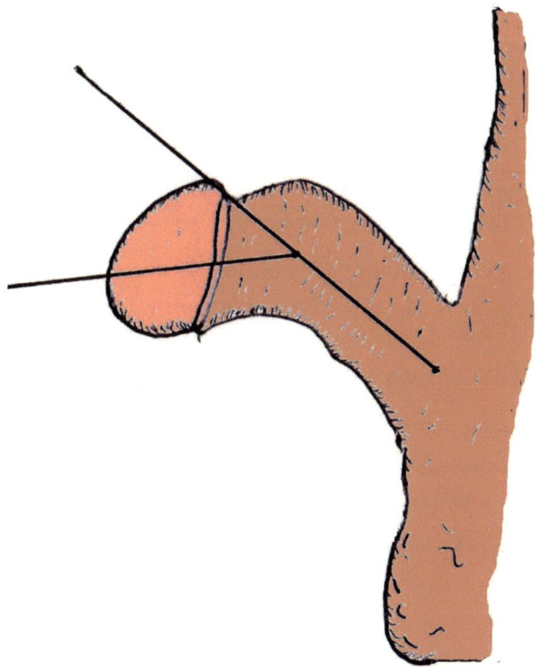

Figure 2. Measurement of the angle of penile curvature.

treatment proposals followed along the next centuries. The Portuguese Amatus Lusitanus (1511–1568) is usually credited as the first to carve a tunnel between the glans and the ectopical meatus. An illustrious patient was King Henry II of France, who presented with a chordee and underwent some kind of procedure in the hands of royal surgeon Jean Fernel. During the eighteenth century, Morgagni compared the condition to the penile groove of turtles and questioned an association between hypospadias and infertility.

The bulk of current techniques derive from conceptual improvements of the nineteenth century. Bouisson proposed a scrotal skin flap to create the inferior wall of the missing urethral segment in 1861. In 1869, Thiersch described tubularised skin grafts as a means to create a neourethra in epispadias (another unrelated urethral malformation). In 1874, Théophile Anger adapted this technique to obtain a successful correction of a penoscrotal hypospadias. In 1880, Duplay described a two-stage repair that included the correction of chordee as the first stage and the urethral reconstruction by means of local flaps from the penile ventral skin as a second stage. Nove-Josserand was the first surgeon to describe free skin grafts to create a neourethra in scrotal hypospadias in 1897.

Former milestones to be cited usually include the works by Matthieu (a flap from proximal skin with parallel sutured lines, 1932), Nesbitt (a technique to treat congenital curvature using fundoplication of the tunica albuginea, 1941), Mustardé (a large flap of perimeatal skin combined with a 'V' incision of the glans, 1965), Duckett [Meatal advancement and glanuloplasty (MAGPI) procedure—1981], Koyanagi (a technique for the more complex scrotal cases, 1984) and Snodgrass (an incision of the tubularised urethral plate, 1994). A great number of surgeons have contributed to this field in order to achieve an acceptable correction to any kind of hypospadias and any claim for 'a new concept' is difficult to prove.

3. Incidence, aetiology and associated malformations

Hypospadias is a common congenital malformation. A nationwide study from Taiwan [4] for the period from 1997 to 2008 has shown a mean incidence of 3.38 per 1000 live male births. A recent series from Sweden [5] has shown an increase from 4.5 cases per 1000 live male births (1973–1989) to 8 per 1000 live male births (1990–2009).

Fortunately, there is a higher incidence of the less severe variants of the condition. Thus, a Dutch series [6] has shown how 59% of hypospadias are anterior (glanular and coronal), 29% are middle (penile) and 12% are posterior (penoscrotal, scrotal and perineal).

Urethral closing is controlled by androgen receptors that bind to dihydrotestosterone. 5-alpha reductase II catalyses the conversion from testosterone to dihydrotestosterone. Most authors mention a multifactorial aetiology and a putative influence on genes that control androgen metabolism. Endocrine disruptors as anti-androgenic substances, hormones or environmental pollutants are heavily suspected as important factors in the pathogenesis of hypospadias in the prenatal period [7]. It is difficult to extrapolate the findings from animals to human beings, however.

Though some genes have been pointed out as causative factors of hypospadias, not many of them have been examined to the point of allowing unequivocal conclusions. There are contradicting studies about the effects of particular drugs on humans, such as the anti-epileptic valproate or the anti-hystaminic loratadine [8].

Hypospadias is more frequent among children of men who themselves have had hypospadias. The risk also rises for the brothers of children with hypospadias [9, 10].

Undescended testis in variable degrees and inguinal hernia are the most common anomalies seen in boys with hypospadias. The more proximal the hypospadias, the more frequent these anomalies.

Diverticula of the prostatic portion of the urethra are seen in severe proximal forms. Infection is a frequent complication of this kind of diverticula and is usually addressed with antibiotic treatment. However, some centres still advise routine explorations of the upper urinary tract in proximal forms [11].

Discovery of intersex states is extremely rare but a karyotype is recommended in case of total cryptorchidism, micropenis, penoscrotal transposition (PST) or biphid scrotum [12].

Imperforate anus and myelomeningocele may be associated with hypospadias. Finally, hypospadias may be part of some complex entities such as McKusick-Kaufman syndrome, Brachmann-de Lange syndrome, Fryns syndrome, Pallister-Hall syndrome, Smith-Lemli-Opitz syndrome, Rapp-Hodgkin syndrome, Marden-Walker syndrome or fronto-facio-nasal dysplasia [13].

4. General surgical principles

4.1. Age for intervention

Technical advances allow operating earlier than in previous decades. Many surgeons advocate intervening in the first 2 years of life for minor distal forms. On the other hand, because increased penile size minimises the risk of producing undesired damage, complicated proximal forms are usually postponed. There is broad consensus to have all procedures done before compulsory school age at 4–5 years with the aim of avoiding psychosocial issues as bullying and comparison with peers [14].

4.2. Optical magnification

Most surgeons think of magnification loupes as a minimal requisite for this kind of surgery; some of them even favour the use of the surgical microscope. Magnification makes the surgeon aware of the importance of minor vessels. In any case, it minimises the rate of complications and it is indispensable in infants and toddlers.

4.3. Instruments and sutures

Many of the instruments used in hypospadias surgery (Castroviejo needle holders, palpebral retractors, microsurgical pincettes) are similar to the ones used in ophthalmic surgery. Depending on centres and individuals, there are some variations but most surgeons apply absorbable polyglactin, polyglycolic acid or monofilament polydioxanone sutures for closing of the neourethra. Nylon or polypropylene are only used in skin sutures and removed after 10–14 days. Surgical calibre of these materials usually varies between 5/0 and 7/0.

4.4. Artificial erection

Introduced in the 1970s [15], the injection of saline solution facilitates correct appreciation of the chordee during the procedure. Some surgeons use it as an ancillary diagnostic procedure before planning an ultimate corrective operation.

4.5. Interposed tissue between skin suture and urethra and biological adhesives

Also starting in the 1970s [16], several techniques have been described to add an extra protective layer of tissue: de-epithelised skin, external spermatic fascia, Buck's fascia, tunica vaginalis or most usually dartos fascia flaps. These procedures decrease significatively the rate of postoperative fistulas [17]. Mobilisation of the dartos muscle over the repair allows 'waterproofing'. Some surgeons use fibrin glue before suturing the final skin layer.

4.6. Haemostasis

As a precaution to prevent undesired burns of the thin penile structures, most surgeons favour bipolar diathermy.

It is generally accepted that using a transient tourniquet to operate in an almost bloodless field eases visualisation and shortens procedure time. (Needless to say, the surgical team must pay attention not to forget tourniquet removal before dressing at the end of the operation.)

4.7. Intraoperative local anaesthesia

A penile block before the end of the operation, using bupivacaine, diminishes pain and the risk of dangerous manipulations of the dressing. Moreover, due to the extensive use of penile block, some minor procedures can be performed as ambulatory day-surgery.

4.8. Catheter drainage

Catheters divert the pressure on the suture zone during the immediate postoperative period. They allow bladder voiding in case of clotting or spasm. As they should be least reactive, silicone is the most favoured catheter or stent material. Catheters and stents provide a priceless protection in middle and proximal hypospadias. Bladder spasm can be reduced by using oxybutynin.

4.9. Dressings

Confection of a mildly compressive dressing deserves special attention at the end of the procedure. A certain degree of pressure is needed to maintain haemostasis and diminish local oedema. A modern trend promotes abstention of any kind of dressing [18]. In any case, all eventual dressings should be non-adhesive to prevent unwanted tearing at the moment of removal.

5. Common surgical procedure

More than 300 techniques have been described for the correction of the diverse types of hypospadias. This great number probably reflects that no single technique can provide an answer to all situations. The average hypospadias surgeon concentrates on mastering a basic arsenal with a certain number of flexible options. Complicated presentations may need complex grafts of mucosa collected from the bladder (introduced by Memmelaar in 1947 [19]) or buccal cavity (first performed by Sapezhko in the nineteenth century [20]).

5.1. The chordee

Correction of chordee should precede any hypospadias surgery to estimate the real length of the straightened urethra (**Figure 3**). A common classification includes four types. Type I is an 'easy' skin tethering. Type II includes a fibrotic fascia. Type III involves corporal disproportion. Type IV consists of a true urethral tethering [21]. The chordee may appear isolated without hypospadias. All fibrous vestiges running along the penile shaft from glans to meatus must be carefully dissected to avoid damage to the urethral plate and the cavernous bodies. Many surgeons prefer a two-stage repair in cases of hypospadias with severe chordee.

http://dx.doi.org/10.5772/intechopen.69924

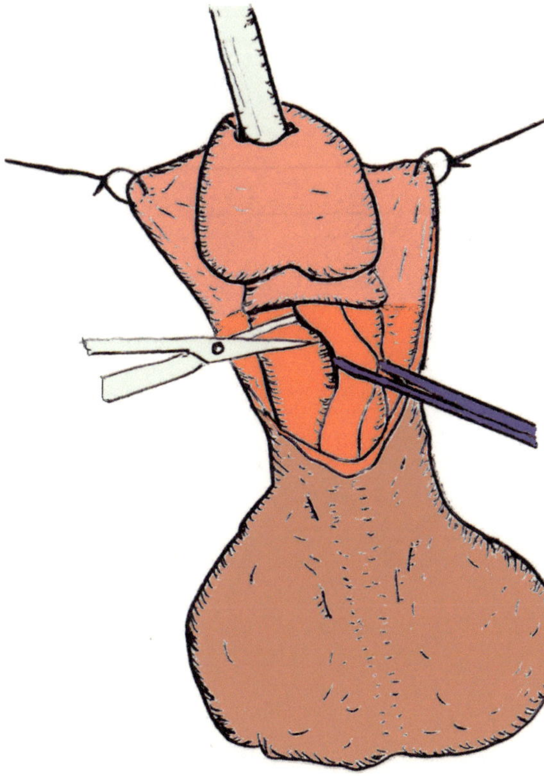

Figure 3. Dissection of a chordee without hypospadias.

5.2. Meatal advancement and glanuloplasty (MAGPI)

The MAGPI technique was described by Duckett in 1981 [22]. It may be useful in the more distal types of hypospadias without chordee that present good skin quality. After liberating the ventral skin, the surgeon performs a triangular suprameatal incision from the point where the new meatus is intended. The centre of the hypospadic meatus is sutured to the vertex of the triangle in order to achieve ascension. The preputial frenulum is simulated by suturing in an inverted 'V', the edges of the missing balanopreputial groove (**Figure 4**).

5.3. Mathieu procedure

Though described by Mathieu in 1932 [23], it bears a strong resemblance to previous operations and has undergone subtle modifications and refinements by surgeons as Gibbons, Devine, Horton, Barcat or van der Meulen to adapt to diverse situations. When the meatus lies subcoronal (or even in the most distal third of the penile shaft), this technique uses a flap of the perimeatal skin to create the missing wall of the urethra in a tubularised way (**Figure 5**).

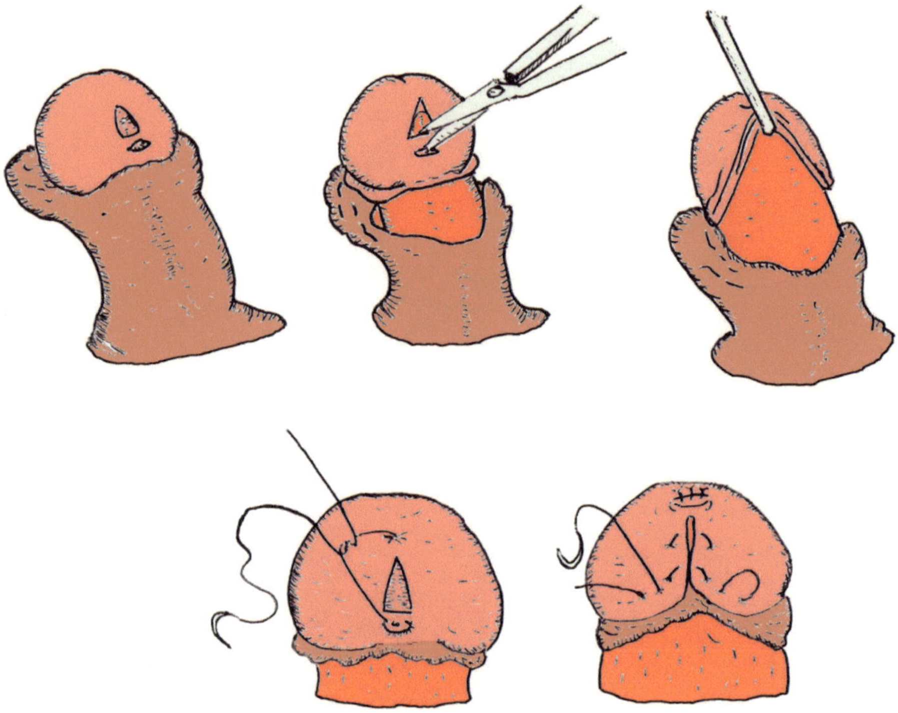

Figure 4. The initial stage and four different phases in the MAGPI technique.

5.4. Byars procedure and Snodgrass adaptation

As described in 1955 [24], this technique is still used on penoscrotal or proximal third types. It is inspired by the concepts of Thiersch and Duplay. The incised edges of the open urethral plate are sewn together and tubularised (**Figure 6**). As usual, there are many variations to this technique.

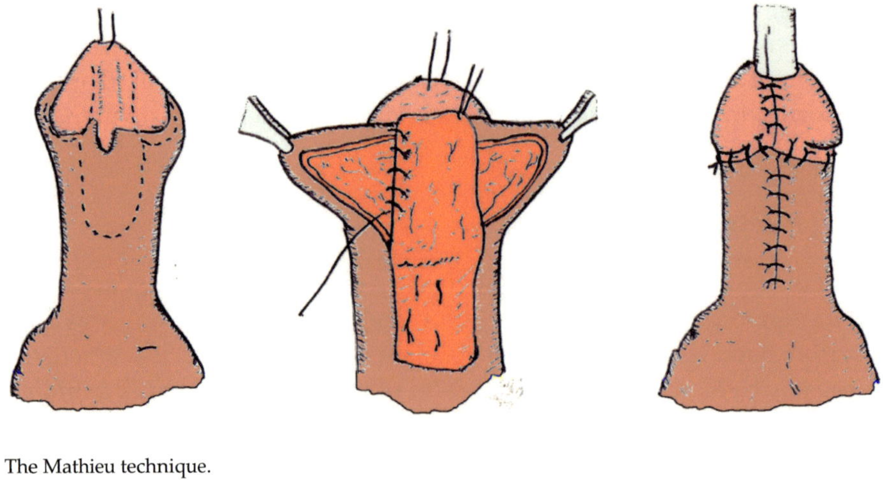

Figure 5. The Mathieu technique.

http://dx.doi.org/10.5772/intechopen.69924

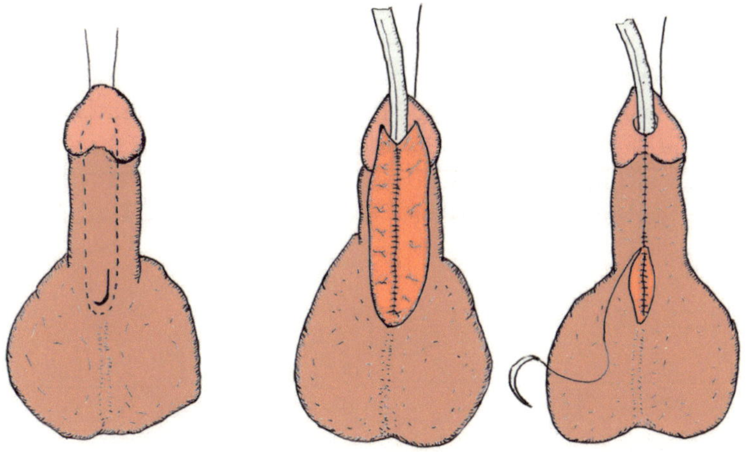

Figure 6. Different stages of the Byars procedure.

Warren Snodgrass introduced a substantial variation [25] that is now becoming the most usual procedure in any kind of hypospadias. He proposed a longitudinal incision of the urethral plate all along the midline. This incision allows easier approaching of the edges of the open urethral plate (**Figure 7**).

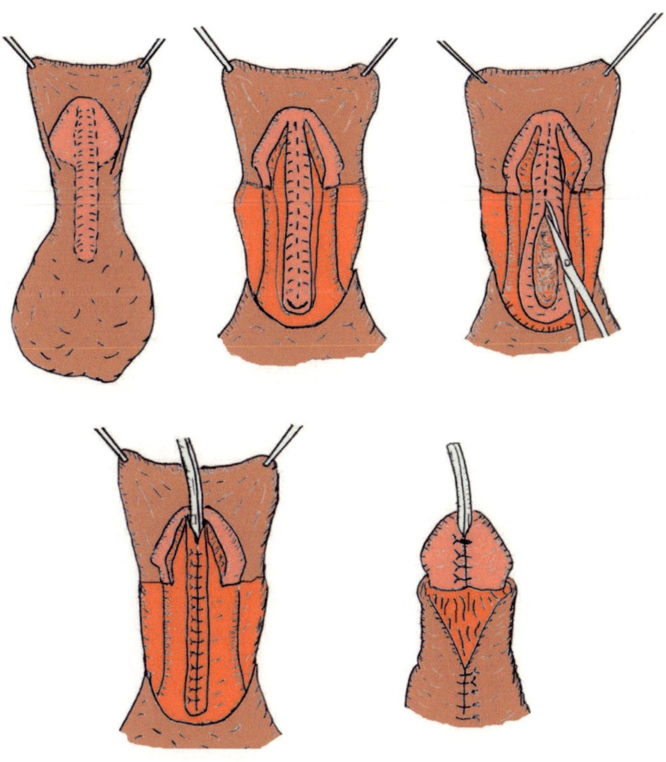

Figure 7. Longitudinal transection of the urethral plate in the Snodgrass procedure.

5.5. Island flap techniques

These are delicate procedures that involve the crafting of a new urethra by using the foreskin [26, 27]. The vascularisation of the preputial flap stems from the basis of the penis and must be preserved to avoid flap necrosis and failure (**Figure 8**). The size of the flap is precisely measured having in sight an undesired retraction (when too short) or diverticula (when too wide). There are different available options for the pedicle.

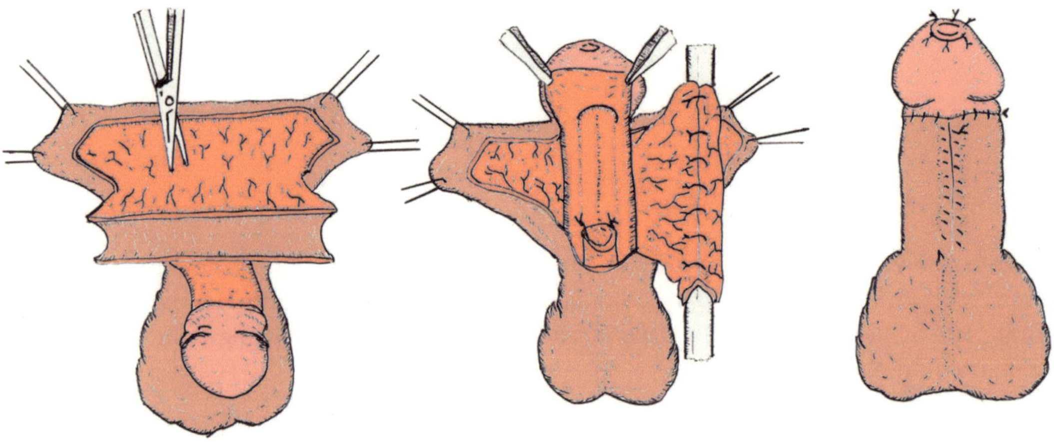

Figure 8. Different stages in the Duckett island flap procedure.

6. Penoscrotal transposition

Penoscrotal transposition (PST) represents a rare congenital abnormality of external genitalia in which the scrotum is positioned superiorly or anteriorly in relation to the penis (**Figure 9**). It includes a large spectrum of anomalies, ranging from the mild bifid scrotum form to the complete penoscrotal transposition (CPST) where the scrotum is located cephalic to the penis [28].

Usually patients present other associated anomalies. Hypospadias, chordee and renal dysplasia as well as anal abnormalities are frequently associated in most patients. Cardiac, gastrointestinal, craniofacial, skeletal and central nervous system malformations have to be ruled out in most severe cases of CPST. Aetiology remains uncertain. A genetic background finds the largest consensus in literature. It is probably linked to an abnormal genital tubercle development around the fifth to sixth week of gestation which might affect the migration and fusion of the scrotum.

Prenatal diagnosis of PST is difficult but it should be considered in the differential diagnosis when ambiguous genitalia or a major urogenital abnormality is suspected on the ultrasound [29].

http://dx.doi.org/10.5772/intechopen.69924

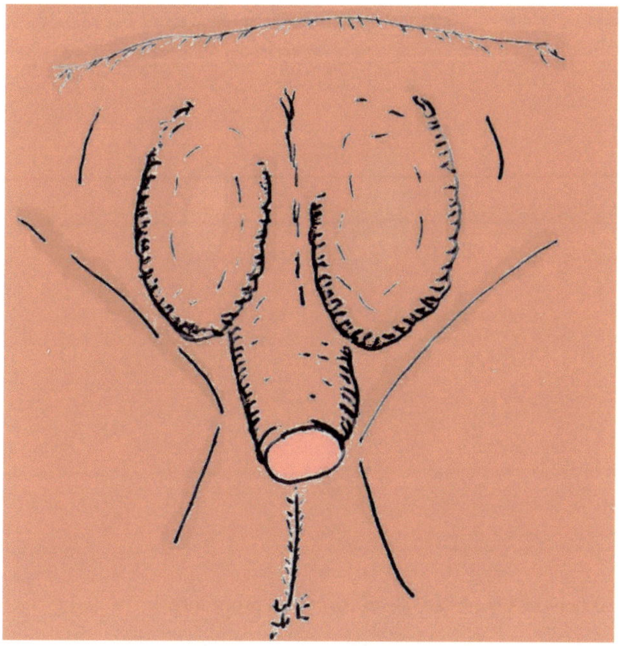

Figure 9. A moderate degree of complete penoscrotal transposition.

Surgical correction is challenging and is usually performed around the 15th–18th month of birth. The size of the phallus and its potential to develop into a sexually satisfactory penis at puberty should be carefully evaluated before surgery. Reassignment to female gender may even be a prudent therapeutic option in a small number of extreme penoscrotal transposition cases due to the unsatisfactory results obtained with penile repositioning and reconstruction [30].

Repairs of penoscrotal transposition rely on the creation of rotational flaps to mobilise the scrotum downwards or transpose the penis to a neo meatus created in the skin of the mons pubis. All procedures entail a complete circular incision around the root of the penis. This usually results in severe and massive oedema of the penile skin, which delays correction of the associated hypospadias and increases the incidence of complications. The skin vascularity and lymphatics may be impaired by the designed incision.

Several surgical techniques are described in the literature for the incomplete PST. The modified Glenn-Anderson [31] techniques are commonly used. In these techniques, the two halves of the scrotum are completely mobilised as a rotational flap and relocated in the right position. The penis can be transposed to a neo hole created in the skin of the mons pubis. To reduce the incidence of oedema of the penile skin consequent upon a circular incision around the root of the penis, Saleh suggests to maintain the penile skin connected to the skin of the lower abdomen by a small strip of skin (**Figure 10**); thus, aids in obtaining a good outcome [32].

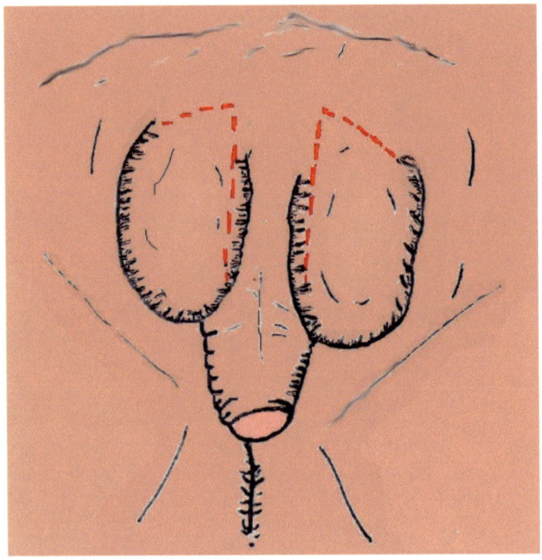

Figure 10. Design of scrotal flaps in a modified Glenn-Anderson procedure.

7. Complications

Many years ago, operating on hypospadias was said to be a sure way to ruin one's reputation in a paediatric department. Complications such as fistulas are unavoidable but fortunately there is remarkable improvement in this area when the above-mentioned general principles are routinely applied [33, 34]. Diverticula are less frequent when appropriate planning is carried out. Skin flap (or even glans!) necrosis and persistent chordee are becoming very rare complications.

7.1. Infection

Perioperative antibiotics may help to reduce the risk of infection, especially with indwelling catheters and adult patients.

7.2. Haemorrhage in the early postoperative period

Usually, it may be prevented with appropriate dressings and non-adherent materials. Instructing the parents and a correct postoperative analgesia would prevent the child to scrub the area.

7.3. Fistulas

Urethrocutaneous fistulas arise from the suture line of the crafted neourethra in all series but their proportion is reported to be from 3 to 20%. Fortunately, this incidence is far from the high values (as much as 45%) observed 40 years ago [35, 36]. Higher fistulisation rates are observed after tubulised free grafts. The most common causes of fistulisation include ischaemia, infection, intolerance to the suture material, distal obstruction to the urine outflow and poor surgical technique. Most teams prefer a waiting period of 6 months before any reoperation. A little number of small early fistulas seems to heal spontaneously. When repairing a fistula, a well-vascularised layer should cover the area (**Figure 11**).

7.4. Stenosis

Most cases of narrow urethra may be treated by dilation in the first preoperative months. Complicated cases may require a new operation that may involve mucosal grafts.

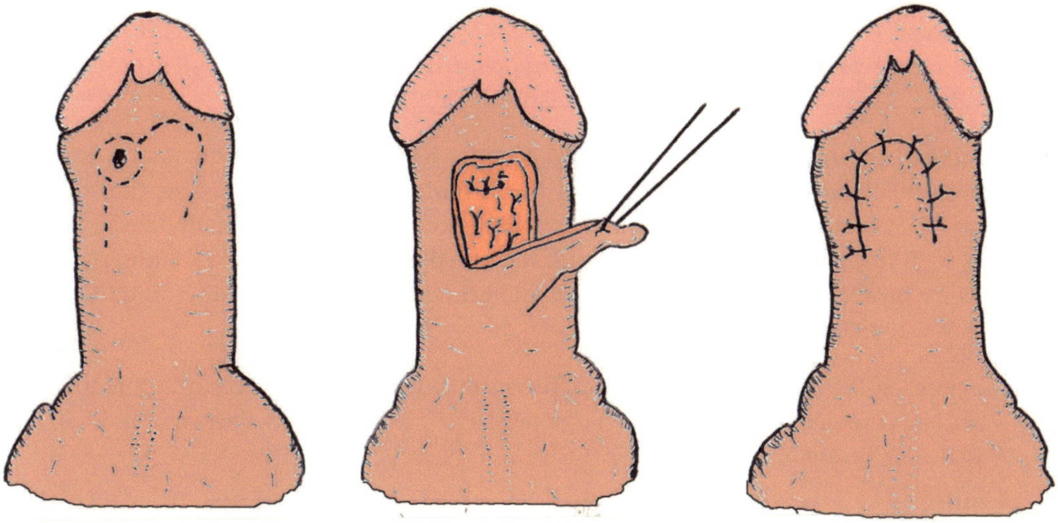

Figure 11. Closing of urethral fistula with a rotating flap.

Author details

Wenceslao M. Calonge[1]* and Gianluca Sapino[2]

*Address all correspondence to: wcalonge@yahoo.es

1 Department of Surgery, Établissements Hospitaliers du Nord Vaudois, Switzerland

2 Department of Plastic, Reconstructive and Aesthetic Surgery, Azienda Ospedaliero–Universitaria di Modena, Italy

References

[1] Hauben DJ. The history of hypospadias. Acta Chirurgica Plastica. 1984;**26**:196-199

[2] Smith ED. The history of hypospadias. Pediatric Surgery International. 1997;**12**:81-85

[3] Thomas DFM. Hypospadiology: Science and surgery. British Journal of Urology International. 2004;**93**:470-473

[4] Huang WY, Chen YF, Guo YJ, Lan CF, Chang HC, Chen SC, Huang KH. Epidemiology of hypospadias and treatment trends in Taiwan: A nationwide study. Journal of Urology. 2011;**185**(4):1449-1454

[5] Nordenvall AS, Frisén L, Nordenström A, Lichtenstein P, Nordenskjöld A. A population-based nationwide study of hypospadias in Sweden, 1973-2009: Incidence and risk factors. J Urol. 2014 Mar;**191**(3):783-789

[6] van Rooij IA, van der Zanden LF, Brouwers MM, Knoers NV, Feitz WF, Roeleveld N. Risk factors for different phenotypes of hypospadias: Results from a Dutch case-control study. British Journal of Urology International. 2013;**112**(1):121-128

[7] Wolf C, Lambright C, Mann P, Price M, Cooper RL, Ostby J, Gray LE. Administration of potentially antiandrogenic pesticides (procymidone, linuron, iprodione, chlozolinate, p,p′-DDE, and ketoconazole) and toxic substances (dibutyl- and diethylhexyl phthalate, PCB 169, and ethane dimethane sulphonate) during sexual differentiation produces diverse profiles of reproductive malformations in the male rat. Toxicology and Industrial Health. 1999;**15**(1-2):94-118

[8] Carmichael SL, Shaw GM, Lammer EJ. Environmental and genetic contributors to hypospadias: A review of the epidemiologic evidence. Birth Defects Research and Clinical Molecular Teratology. 2012;**94**(7):499-510

[9] Angerpointner TA. Hypospadias – genetics, epidemiology and other possible aetiological influences. Zeitschrift Kinderchirurgie (European Journal of Pediatric Surgery). 1984;**39**:112-118

[10] Wilcox DT, Mouriquand PDE. Hypospadias. In: Thomas DFM, Duffy PG, Rickwood AMK, editors. Essentials of pediatric urology. London: Informa Healthcare; 2008. pp. 213-232

[11] Cerasaro TS, Brock WA, Kaplan GW. Upper urinary tract anomalies with congenital hypospadias: Is screening necessary? Journal of Urology. 1986;**135**:537-538

[12] McAleer IM, Kaplan GW. Is routine karyotyping necessary in the evaluation of hypospadias and cryptorchidism? Journal of Urology. 2001;**165**:2029-2031

[13] Boehmer AL, Nijman RJ, Lammers BA. Etiological studies of severe or familial hypospadias. Journal of Urology. 2001;**165**:1246-1254

[14] Hadidi AT. Principles of hypospadias surgery. In: Hadidi AT, Azmy AF, editors. Hypospadias Surgery. An Illustrated Guide. Berlin: Springer; 2004. pp. 99-105

[15] Gittes RF, McLaughlin III AP. Injection technique to induce penile erection. Urology. 1974;**4**:473-474

[16] Smith D. A de-epithelialized overlap flap technique in the repair of hypospadias. British Journal of Plastic Surgery. 1973;**26**:106-114

[17] Gapany C, Grasset N, Tercier S, Ramseyer P, Frey P, Meyrat BJ. A lower fistula rate in hypospadias surgery. Journal of Pediatric Urology. 2007:**3**(5):395-397

[18] van Savage JG, Palanca LG, Slaughenhoupt BL. A prospective randomized trial of dressings versus no dressings for hypospadias repair. Journal of Urology. 2000;**164**:981-983

[19] Memmelaar J. Use of bladder mucosa in a one-stage repair of hypospadias. Journal of Urology. 1947;**58**(1):68-73

[20] Korneyev I, Ilyin D, Schultheiss D, Chapple C. The first oral mucosal graft urethroplasty was carried out in the 19th century: The pioneering experience of Kirill Sapezhko (1857-1928). European Urology. 2012;**62**(4):624-627

[21] Donnahoo KK, Cain MP, Pope JC, Casale AJ, Keating MA, Adams MC, Rink RC. Etiology, management and surgical complications of congenital chordee without hypospadias. Journal of Urology. 1998;**160**(3)2:1120-1122

[22] Duckett JW. MAGPY (meatal advancement and glanuloplasty), a procedure for subcoronal hypospadias. Urologic Clinics of North America. 1981;**5**:513-520

[23] Mathieu MP. Traitement en un temps de l'hypospadias balanique ou yuxtabalanique. Journal de Chirurgie. 1932;**39**:481-486

[24] Byars LT. A technique for consistently satisfactory repair of hypospadias. Surgical Gynecology and Obstetrics. 1955;**100**(2):184-190

[25] Snodgrass WT. Tubularized incised plate hypospadias repair. In: Frank D, Gearhart JP, Snyder HM, editors. Operative Pediatric Urology. London: Churchill Livingstone; 2002. pp. 161-164

[26] Duckett JW. The island flap technique for hypospadias repair. Urologic Clinics of North America. 1981;**8**:503

[27] Duckett JW. Hypospadias repair. In: Frank D, Gearhart JP, Snyder HM, editors. Operative Pediatric Urology. London: Churchill Livingstone; 2002. pp. 149-160

[28] Avolio L, Karmarkar SJ, Martucciello G. Complete penoscrotal transposition. Urology. 2006;**67**(6):1287

[29] Sexton P, Thomas JT, Petersen S, Brown N, Arms JE, Bryan J, Harraway J, Gardener G. Complete penoscrotal transposition: Case report and review of the literature. Fetal Diagnosis and Therapy. 2015;**37**(1):70-74

[30] Naren SD, Soren C, Subbarao PV. Penoscrotal transposition: A case report. Indian Journal of Surgery. 2013;**75**(1):64-65

[31] Saleh A. Correction of incomplete penoscrotal transposition by a modified Glenn-Anderson technique. African Journal of Paediatric Surgery. 2010;**7**(3):181-184

[32] Glenn JF, Anderson EE. Surgical correction of incomplete penoscrotal transposition. Journal of Urology. 1973;**110**(5):603-605

[33] Shapiro SR. Complications in hypospadias repair. Journal of Urology. 1973;**131**:518-522

[34] Retik AB, Keating MA, Mandell J. Complications of hypospadias surgery. Urologic Clinics of North America. 1981;**8**:223-236

[35] Horton CE, Devine CJ. Urethral fistula. In: Horton CE, editor. Plastic and reconstructive surgery of the genital area. Boston: Little & Brown Co; 1973. pp. 397-403

[36] Baskins LS. Hypospadias. In: Stringer MD, Oldham KT, Mouriquand PDE, editors. Paediatric Surgery and Urology. Long-term Outcomes. Cambridge; Cambridge University Press; 2006. pp. 611-620